Interdisciplinary Statistics

MEASUREMENT ERROR and MISCLASSIFICATION in STATISTICS and EPIDEMIOLOGY

Impacts and Bayesian Adjustments

CHAPMAN & HALL/CRC
Interdisciplinary Statistics Series

Series editors: N. Keiding, B. Morgan, T. Speed, P. van der Heijden

Interdisciplinary Statistics

MEASUREMENT ERROR and MISCLASSIFICATION in STATISTICS and EPIDEMIOLOGY

Impacts and Bayesian Adjustments

Paul Gustafson

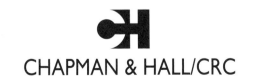

CHAPMAN & HALL/CRC

A CRC Press Company
Boca Raton   London   New York   Washington, D.C.

Library of Congress Cataloging-in-Publication Data

Gustafson, Paul.
  Measurement error and misclassification in statistics and epidemiology : impacts and
  Bayesian adjustments / Paul Gustafson
          p.   cm. (Chapman & Hall/CRC Interdisciplinary Statistics Series; 13)
  Includes bibliographical references and index.
  ISBN 1-58488-335-9
  1. Error analysis (Mathematics). 2. Sequential analysis. 3. Bayesian statistical decision
  theory. I. Title.

QA275.G93 2003
511′.43—dc22   2003047290

Visit the CRC Press Web site at www.crcpress.com

© 2004 by Chapman & Hall/CRC

No claim to original U.S. Government works
International Standard Book Number 1-58488-335-9
Library of Congress Card Number 2003047290
Printed in the United States of America 1 2 3 4 5 6 7 8 9 0
Printed on acid-free paper

To Reka, Joseph, Lucas, and Anna

Contents

Preface

One of the most fundamental tasks in statistical science is to understand the relationship between some *explanatory variables* and a *response* or *outcome* variable. This book discusses problems and solutions associated with statistical analysis when an explanatory variable is *mismeasured*. That is, the variable in question cannot be observed, though a rough surrogate for it can be measured. While it is tempting to simply 'plug-in' this surrogate and proceed as usual, one must be mindful that scientific interest will be focussed on how the actual but unobservable variable impacts the response variable. When the variable in question is continuous in nature, this sort of scenario is often referred to as involving *errors-in-variables*, *errors-in-covariables*, or simply *measurement error*. When the explanatory variable in question is categorical, often *misclassification* is the term used. We deliberately use *mismeasurement* to encompass both scenarios.

Mismeasurement of explanatory variables is quite common in many scientific areas where statistical modelling is brought to bear. While the statistical discussion and development herein is general, our examples are drawn from biostatistics and epidemiology. In these fields, statistical models are often applied to explanatory variables which reflect human *exposure* of one kind or another. Many exposures of medical interest cannot be measured very precisely at the level of the individual, with prime examples being exposures to indoor and outdoor pollutants, and exposures based on food and drug intakes. In recognition of this problem, much of the literature on mismeasured explanatory variables has a biostatistical or epidemiological focus.

Perhaps it is easiest to characterize this book in terms of what it is not. First, it is not a textbook, nor is it strictly a research monograph. Rather, it presents a mix of expository material and research-oriented material. However, much of the expository material is presented in a new light, with nuances and emphases that differ from those of existing references. Second, this book is not comprehensive. The statistical literature on adjusting for mismeasurement is surprisingly large, and also somewhat unwieldy. I do not claim to cover all facets of it. Rather, the book focusses on some of the main ideas, and then delves selectively into more advanced topics. The choice of topics reflects my own views on what are interesting, relevant, and topical issues in understanding and adjusting for mismeasurement.

If asked to identify novel aspects of this book, I would start by noting its dual treatment of mismeasurement in both continuous and categorical variables. Historically there seems to be a somewhat artificial divide, with the continuous case dealt with in the statistics and biostatistics literature, and the categorical case dealt with in the epidemiology literature. In other statistical research areas the distinction between continuous and categorical explanatory variables is much less important. This book aims to draw the two topics together as much as possible, and to be of interest to both the (bio)statistics community, and at least the more quantitative subset of the epidemiology community.

A second novel feature of the book is that all the statistical modelling to adjust for mismeasurement is done within the *Bayesian* paradigm for statistical inference. This paradigm provides a conceptually simple and general approach to statistical analysis. The Bayesian approach has received much attention over the last decade or so, now that powerful *Markov chain Monte Carlo* computational algorithms are available to implement Bayesian methods in complex scenarios. While a number of research articles have demonstrated the utility of the Bayesian approach in adjusting for mismeasurement, to date there has not been an overarching reference on this topic.

A third noteworthy feature of the book is that a slightly sceptical 'wrong-model' view of the world is adopted in many places. In contrast to much of the literature, when considering the impact of unchecked mismeasurement it is usually not assumed that the postulated statistical models are correct. And there is some emphasis on how adjustments for mismeasurement will fare when the entertained models are not correct. The famous adage of G.E.P. Box that "all models are wrong, but some are useful" is quite central to much of the book's developments.

The book should be accessible to graduate students, practitioners, and researchers in Statistics and Biostatistics, and to Epidemiologists with particular interest in quantitative methods. Much of the mathematical detail in each chapter is collected in a final section, with the goal of making the main body of the chapter more accessible. As well, there is a largely self-contained Appendix introducing the main ideas of Bayesian analysis and Markov chain Monte Carlo algorithms, for the sake of readers without previous exposure to these topics.

I am grateful to a number of organizations and people for help in bringing this book to fruition. I thank the Natural Sciences and Engineering Research Council of Canada and the Canadian Institutes of Health Research for research grant support. I thank Kirsty Stroud, Jasmin Naim, and Jamie Sigal at Chapman and Hall/CRC for their help, and particularly for their patience when I adopted the typical professorial interpretation of deadlines. I thank all my colleagues in the Department of Statistics at U.B.C. for collectively providing such a convivial environment for academic pursuits, with particular thanks to Nhu Le for venturing into the mismeasurement world with me, and to Jim Zidek for suggesting I write this book in the first place. Above all, I thank my wife, and my children—of whom there were two when I started writing and three when I finished. They were all much better sports about this endeavour than they ought to have been!

Guide to Notation

Some commonly used notation is as follows.

AF	attenuation factor
Y	outcome or response variable (continuous or binary)
X	unobservable continuous explanatory variable of interest
X^*	observable surrogate for X
V	unobservable binary explanatory variable of interest
V^*	observable surrogate for V
Z	other observable explanatory variables (of any type)
θ_M	all the parameters in the measurement model
τ^2	the variance of X^* given X in the measurement model
θ_R	all the parameters in the response model
β	regression coefficients in the response model
θ_{E1}	all the parameters in the conditional exposure model
α	regression coefficients in the conditional exposure model
(SN, SP)	sensitivity and specificity for V^* as a surrogate for V
(p, q)	more compact notation for sensitivity and specificity
$(\tilde{p}, \tilde{q})$	(incorrectly) assumed values of (p, q)
r_i	prevalence of binary exposure in i-th population
Ψ	odds-ratio
ψ	log odds-ratio

CHAPTER 1

Introduction

The quintessential statistical task is to understand or 'learn' the relationship between an outcome variable Y and an explanatory variable X, having observed both variables simultaneously for a number of study units. Often in biostatistical and epidemiological investigations the study units are people, the outcome variable is health-related, and the explanatory variable reflects an *exposure* of some kind. This book is concerned with consequences and remedies if in fact the explanatory variable cannot be measured very precisely. Specifically, sometimes a rough or *surrogate* variable X^* is recorded, rather than X itself. Whereas the scientific goal is to understand the relationship between X and Y, the available data consist of measurements of X^* and Y (and usually other variables as well). This book focusses on how misleading it is to ignore this 'disconnect' by analyzing the data as if they were precisely measured, and on how to generate statistical inferences that reflect or adjust for the mismeasurement at play. We start by giving some examples where it is necessary to rely on surrogate explanatory variables. While such contexts abound in many subject areas where statistical methods are used, we focus on scenarios from medical research.

1.1 Examples of Mismeasurement

Many variables of interest to medical researchers as possible culprits in the development of disease are difficult to measure on individuals. Intakes of various foods and drugs are prime examples, as are exposures to ambient entities such as airborne pollutants, radiation, and magnetic fields. To give some specific examples we mention three scenarios taken from the recent epidemiological literature.

Brown, Kreiger, Darlington and Sloan (2001) investigate the common scenario where X is average daily caffeine intake, but X^* is based on the self-reported average cups of coffee consumed. In particular, X^* is the average number of cups per day reported by a subject on a questionnaire, multiplied by the amount of caffeine in a 'standard' cup of coffee, i.e., a cup of typical size and strength. On biological grounds the relationship between an outcome Y and X is of much more interest than the relationship between Y and X^*. Brown *et al.* conduct a study to assess how closely X^* and X tend to agree, and give some implications for statistical analysis in hypothetical scenarios with a strong association between X and Y. In particular, study participants are questioned about typical intake of a variety of caffeine-containing products, leading to a demonstration that X^* based on coffee alone often vastly underestimates X. The authors then recommend that in practice questionnaires include queries about tea and cola consumption, as well as coffee consumption. It should be noted, however, that this is far from the end of the story. In this scenario mismeasurement also arises because participants have imperfect recall when completing questionnaires, and because some subjects will have a systematic tendency to consume cups of coffee with caffeine content higher or lower than that of a standard cup. Thus even very detailed questionnaires are likely to yield substantial mismeasurement of caffeine intake.

More generally, nutritional intakes are exposure variables of considerable interest in medical studies, while also being difficult to measure. In studies with large numbers of subjects, resource limitations might only allow for use of a *food-frequency questionnaire* (FFQ), on which subjects self-report the frequency with which they consume specific foods. Sometimes, however, it is possible to make more precise measurements on a small subset of study subjects. For instance, Rosner and Gore (2001) consider the Nurses' Health Study, where a FFQ was administered to about 89,000 subjects, with additional detailed measurements obtained for about 170 of these subjects. The subset of subjects for whom both measurements are made is referred to as the *validation sample*, while those for whom only the rougher measurement is made constitute the main sample. In the present scenario the more detailed measurements are based on a weighed diet record, whereby subjects weigh and record what they eat in real-time over a short period. We can regard $X = (X_1, \ldots, X_J)$ as the intake of a J different foods for a given subject according to the weighed diet record, while $X^* = (X_1^*, \ldots, X_J^*)$ are the analogous intakes as determined from the FFQ. Rosner and Gore demonstrate that the precision with which X_j can be predicted from X^* varies considerably across j, i.e., the FFQ works better for some foods than others. A very important point is that even a small validation sample gives some basis for guessing the unobserved values of X from the observed values of X^* in main sample subjects. Thus one sees opportunity to do better than an analysis which simply proceeds by treating X^* as if it were X.

Another general class of variables that are subject to considerable mismeasurement are biochemical variables based on laboratory analysis of human-subject samples. As one example, Bashir, Duffy and Qizilbash (1997) describe a study where the outcome is incidence of minor ischaemic stroke, while the explanatory variables of interest are levels of four haemostatic factors—agents which retard the flow of blood in blood vessels. The study follows a case–control design, comparing a group of subjects who had a minor stroke to a group that did not. Initial blood samples were assayed twice, giving two measurements of the factor levels. Also, one-year follow-up blood samples were obtained for some of the control subjects, and these were also assayed twice. As is typical for biochemical variables, mismeasurement is at play here in two ways. First, there is pure laboratory error which leads to two different numerical measurements for the same blood sample. Second, levels of the haemostatic factors vary somewhat from day-to-day within a given subject. Operationally it makes sense to define the explanatory variable as the subject's average level, but measurement error arises because of the day-to-day fluctuations. Even in the absence of pure laboratory error then, two blood samples taken on different days are not likely to give identical measurements. Bashir *et al.* discuss the implications of both sources of mismeasurement for inference about the relationship between the haemostatic factors and incidence of stroke.

Examples such as these speak to the difficulty in measuring many explanatory variables of interest to medical researchers. Indeed, exposure assessment itself is a very important area of Epidemiology (see, for instance, the book by Armstrong, White and Saracci 1992). In many circumstances, however, substantial mismeasurement will remain no matter how much care and expense is devoted to measuring the variable in question. This behooves us to (i) consider what effect mismeasurement might have on a statistical analysis which simply pretends the surrogate variable X^* is the real explanatory variable X, and (ii) contemplate more refined statistical analysis which acknowledges the difference between the observable X^* and the unobservable X, while retaining an inferential focus on the relationship between X and Y.

1.2 The Mismeasurement Phenomenon

Henceforth an analysis which pretends the surrogate variable is the same as the variable of interest is referred to as *naive*, since it pretends mismeasurement is not manifested. One can glean a sense of how well naive analysis performs with some simple computer-simulated examples. Before doing so, however, we acknowledge an asymmetry in our development. We focus on situations where the explanatory variable X is subject to mismeasurement, and ignore equally realistic scenarios where the outcome variable Y is subject to mismeasurement. The following simulations speak to this seemingly arbitrary choice of focus.

Consider the scatterplot of simulated data displayed in the upper-left panel of Figure 1.1. These data consist of 500 (X, Y) pairs. For completeness we note that the data were simulated from a bivariate normal distribution with both means equal to zero, both variances equal to one, and a correlation coefficient of 0.5. Fitting a standard linear regression to these data gives $0.012 + 0.514X$ as the estimated conditional expectation of Y given X. This fitted regression line is superimposed on the plotted points. In the usual manner we interpret the estimated slope as describing a 0.514 unit change in the average value of Y per one unit change in X. The standard error associated with the slope estimate is 0.037.

Now say that in fact the outcome variable is subject to measurement error, so that Y^* is observed in lieu of Y, where Y^* is obtained by adding 'noise' to Y, without any regard to the X variable. In the present example the noise is taken to have a normal distribution with mean zero and variance one. A scatterplot of the (X, Y^*) pairs appears in the lower-left panel of Figure 1.1, with the fitted linear regression line superimposed. The slope of this line is 0.475, with a standard error of 0.060. It comes as no surprise that the

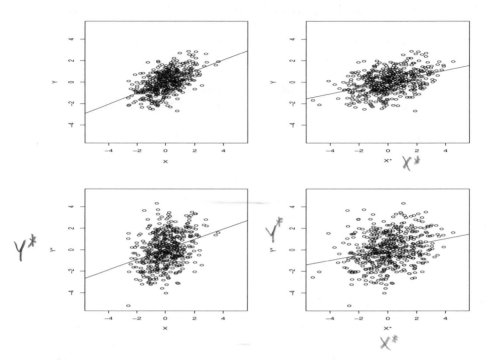

Figure 1.1 *Scatterplots for the example of Section 1.2. Starting at the upper-left and proceeding clockwise we have scatterplots of (X, Y), (X^*, Y), (X^*, Y^*), and (X, Y^*).*

addition of noise to Y does not change the slope estimate greatly, but it does increase the the reported uncertainty in the estimate, i.e., the standard error. Mathematically it is simple to verify that if Y^* is obtained by adding noise to Y, then the conditional expectation of Y^* given X is identically the conditional expectation of Y given X, provided the noise is uncorrelated with X. Thus adding noise to Y does not shift the estimated regression relationship in a systematic manner, though it does increase the inferential uncertainty about the (X, Y) relationship.

In contrast, say X rather than Y is subject to measurement error. The upper-right panel of Figure 1.1 gives a scatterplot of (X^*, Y), where X^* is obtained from X by adding normal noise which is independent of Y. Again the noise itself has mean zero and variance one. Visually the fitted regression line is flatter than that for (X, Y), with an estimated slope of 0.272 and a standard error of 0.027. Moreover it is hard to attribute this difference to chance in any sense. An approximate 95% confidence interval for the population slope of (X, Y) is 0.51 ± 0.07, while a similar interval from the (X^*, Y) regression is 0.27 ± 0.05. Indeed, it is not hard to verify that the conditional expectation of Y given $X^* = a$ and the conditional expectation of Y given $X = a$ are *different* functions of a. Put succinctly, if we are interested in estimating the conditional expectation of Y given X, then adding noise to X imparts a bias, whereas adding noise to Y does not. This explains the common emphasis on mismeasurement of explanatory variables rather than mismeasurement of outcome variables.

For completeness the lower-right panel of Figure 1.1 considers the case of mismeasurement in both variables, i.e., Y^* is regressed on X^*. As might be expected the estimated regression line is close to that obtained when Y is regressed on X^*. Again, adding noise to Y does not impart a systematic change in the estimated regression function.

On the face of it a bias resulting from the mismeasurement described above might seem surprising, as the nature of the mismeasurement itself seems free from bias. In particular, the particular mismeasurement mechanism might be described as both 'blind' and 'fair.' It is blind in the sense of not depending on the outcome variable (formally the distribution of X^* given X and Y does not depend on Y), and it is fair in the sense of not systematically favouring under or over measurement (formally the distribution of X^* given X is symmetric about X). However, in looking at Figure 1.1 one can gain some geometric insight into why an inferential bias results. The impact of adding noise to the X variable is to spread out the point cloud in the horizontal direction while leaving it fixed in the vertical direction. This leads directly to a flatter slope for the regression line. On the other hand, adding noise to Y does not have an analogous effect. Since the regression line is based on minimizing the vertical variation of the points from the line, adding noise to Y does not exert a systematic 'pull' on the line.

In fact, a flattening or *attenuation* in the apparent strength of association between explanatory and outcome variables induced by mismeasurement of the explanatory variable is quite a general phenomenon. To give a simple demonstration that it carries over to categorical variables, consider a binary outcome variable Y and a binary explanatory variable V (throughout the book X and V are reserved as labels for continuous and categorical explanatory variables respectively). Say that (V, Y) values for a sample of 500 subjects are as given on the left side of Table 1.1. In particular, the empirical odds-ratio for this table is 2.68, indicating a strong positive association betwen V and Y. Now say that V cannot be measured precisely, and rather V^* is recorded, where V^* is a noisy version of V. In particular, say that each subject has a 20% chance of V^* differing from V, regardless of the value of Y. A simulated realization of V^* values yields the (V^*, Y) table on the right side of Table 1.1. The empirical odds-ratio for this table is only 2.00. Again the impact of mismeasurement is a weaker estimated relationship between the explanatory and outcome variables. Note that again attenuation is manifested even though the mismeasurement is blind to the outcome variable, and fair in the sense that the chance of mismeasurement is the same whether $V = 0$ or $V = 1$.

Thus far we have suggested that many explanatory variables of interest cannot be measured very well, and we have shown that doing the analysis by pretending the surrogate is actually the variable of interest can lead to biased inferences, not just less precise inferences. These two findings provide a rationale for what is discussed and developed in the remainder of the book.

	$Y = 0$	$Y = 1$		$Y = 0$	$Y = 1$
$V = 0$	378	39	$V^* = 0$	331	34
$V = 1$	65	18	$V^* = 1$	112	23

Table 1.1 *Simulated binary data for* 500 *subjects. Both* (V, Y) *and* (V^*, Y) *tables are given.*

1.3 What is Ahead?

The basic road-map for what is covered in this book is quite simple. Chapters 2 and 3 investigate the properties and performance of naive estimation for mismeasured continuous and categorical variables respectively. In particular, the magnitude of the attenuating bias seen in Figure 1.1 and Table 1.1 is quantified in a variety of realistic scenarios. Much of the literature gives cursory coverage of how well naive estimation performs before moving on to statistical methods which try to reverse the impact of mismeasurement. In contrast, Chapters 2 and 3 take a more detailed and leisurely look at the circumstances which make the attenuation slight or substantial. This material can be regarded as useful for developing intuition about when it is important to try to reverse the impact of mismeasurement.

Having studied the quality of naive inference, Chapters 4 and 5 turn to statistical analysis which aims to 'undo' the impact of mismeasurement. Often this might be referred to as *adjusting, accounting,* or *correcting* for mismeasurement. Again the separate chapters deal with continuous and categorical variables respectively. Examples of such analysis applied to both simulated datasets and real datasets are provided, and a variety of modelling strategies and issues are discussed. A central focus in these chapters is discussion of how much must be assumed or known about the mismeasurement process in order to implement a reasonable analysis which accounts for the mismeasurement.

Chapter 6 concludes the book with a look at three more specialized topics surrounding the impact of mismeasurement and attempts to ameliorate this impact. While the topics are chosen idiosyncratically, collectively they give some idea of the surprising and intricate 'twists and turns' surrounding the mismeasurement of explanatory variables. First, scenarios where a mismeasured binary variable is created from a mismeasured continuous variable are studied. It turns out that such scenarios are quite realistic, and the impact of mismeasurement in this context differs greatly from that of 'ordinary' misclassification. Second, the interplay between model misspecification and mismeasurement is scrutinized. Biased inference may arise because the postulated model for the outcome Y given the unobservable explanatory variable X is incorrect. Interesting connections and contrasts between this bias and the bias due to mismeasurement are seen to arise. Third, close attention is given to the question of how much must be known and understood about the mismeasurement process for a mismeasurement adjustment to be worthwhile. This investigation is based on quantifying the performance of estimation procedures when formally the statistical model at hand is *nonidentifiable.*

As implied by the book's subtitle, the work in Chapters 4 and 5 on adjusting for mismeasurement is undertaken via the Bayesian paradigm for statistical inference. In contrast, other books and review articles on adjusting for mismeasured variables focus almost exclusively on non-Bayesian techniques (Fuller 1987, Walter and Irwig 1987, Chen 1989, Willett 1989, Thomas, Stram and Dwyer 1993, Carroll, Ruppert and Stefanski 1995 Bashir and Duffy 1997). The present author's premise is that the Bayesian handling of unobserved quantities yields a very natural treatment of mismeasurement problems. In particular, the analysis involves aggregating over plausible values of the correct but unobserved variable. While the Bayesian approach has long been recognized as conceptually appealing, computational difficulties have been its historic Achilles' heel. Essentially, high-dimensional mathematical integration is required. The Bayesian approach has become popular in the last decade or so with the advent of new computational algorithms that tackle this integration in an indirect way. In fact, these algorithms originated much earlier in the statistical physics literature, but sustained technology-transfer to the statistical community did not commence until the work of Gelfand and Smith (1990). They introduced the *Gibbs sampling* algorithm to the statistical community, which in turn is a special instance of the class of *Markov chain Monte Carlo* (MCMC) algorithms. Most of the analyses given in Chapters 4 and 5 are implemented via MCMC algorithms. For the sake of readers unfamiliar with the Bayesian paradigm, an Appendix gives a self-contained, skeletal description of Bayesian inference and MCMC algorithms in general.

This book is intended to be neither strictly applied nor strictly theoretical in nature. The example analyses provided are meant to demonstrate what can be accomplished with the general modelling strategies presented. They are not intended as methodologies which can be taken 'off-the-shelf' and applied without modification in new problems. Mismeasurement scenarios tend to be specialized and nuanced, and usually some refinements are required to adapt a given methodology for a particular problem. On the other hand, the book is written with the idea of focussing on issues of general relevance to applied work. The overall tone of the book reflects the author's penchant for topics and issues involving an interplay between statistical theory and application. As well, the text tends to move back and forth between expounding established concepts and delving into areas of current research. This is done with the aim of focussing on the most interesting and relevant ideas, be they old or new.

The computed examples in this book are implemented in the R environment (www.r-project.org), which is standard software in the academic statistics community. Very roughly put, the R environment is an Open Source variant of the S-Plus environment (www.insightful.com). The computer code for the examples is available on the author's website (www.stat.ubc.ca/people/gustaf). Implementing MCMC algorithms in R is relatively easy given the underlying mathematical and statistical functionality of the software. Another good alternative for implementing MCMC which is not pursued here is the BUGS software (www.mrc-bsu.cam.ac.uk/bugs). BUGS has developed into the primary MCMC-specific software package. For problems without unusual features BUGS is ideal, as the user need only specify the modelling details of the problem at hand. The software then determines and runs an appropriate MCMC algorithm. Some of the examples in the book could be readily implemented via BUGS. On the other hand, some of the examples involve 'tricky' application of MCMC, where it is necessary to exert direct control over the algorithmic details. This prompts the choice of R as the implementation platform.

CHAPTER 2

The Impact of Mismeasured Continuous Variables

In the first chapter we gave an intuitive explanation as to how the mismeasurement phenomenon arises, i.e., how measurement error in a continuous explanatory variable typically attenuates the associated regression coefficient. Now we mathematically elucidate this attenuation, first in the simple scenario of Chapter 1 and then in more complex scenarios. There is no attempt yet to adjust estimators to account for measurement error; this is taken up in Chapter 4. Rather, the goal of this chapter is to quantify the degradation of naive inference in various settings. It can be very useful to develop some intuition in this regard, as in some scenarios not enough is known about the mismeasurement process to attempt a formal adjustment.

The majority of the material in this chapter is not new, though arguably it has a wider range and different flavour than other discussions of how well naive estimation performs in the face of measurement error. One notable feature is that most of the present treatment permit a discrepancy between the actual and modelled relationships for the outcome variable in terms of the actual but unobservable explanatory variable. That is, the bias induced by measurement error can be quantified without regard for the extent of model misspecification at hand. In general it is the author's contention that much of the mismeasured variable literature gives short shrift to discussion of how ignoring the mismeasurement affects the quality of inference. In contrast, we take a detailed and leisurely look at when naive estimation does or does not work well before turning our attention to adjustment in Chapter 4.

2.1 The Archetypical Scenario

To return to the scenario described in Chapter 1, say the investigator is interested in the relationship between the continuous response Y and the continuous predictor X, and correctly surmises that $E(Y|X) = \beta_0 + \beta_1 X$ for unknown coefficients β_0 and β_1. However, while Y can be measured correctly, X^* is measured in lieu of X. If the investigator is unaware of this mismeasurement, or chooses to ignore it, he may interpret the estimated coefficients from a linear regression of Y on X^* as describing the relationship of interest between Y and X.

It is straightforward to quantify the damage resulting from this actual or feigned ignorance under some assumptions about the precise predictor X and its imprecise surrogate X^*. Particularly, assume that X has a normal distribution, and say that X^* arises from additive measurement error which is _non-differential_, _unbiased_, and normally distributed. In general mismeasurement is said to be nondifferential if the distribution of the surrogate variable depends only on the actual explanatory variable and not on the reponse variable. Intuitively this can be regarded as a supposition that the mismeasurement arises in a manner which is blind to the outcome variable, so in some sense the problem is limited to one of difficulty in making measurements. Stated more formally, we say the measurement error is nondifferential when X^* and Y are conditionally independent of Y, so that the conditional distribution of $(X^*|X,Y)$ is identically the conditional distribution of $(X^*|X)$. We further restrict to unbiased measurement error, i.e., $E(X^*|X) = X$, and in fact assume a normal distribution with constant variance for the conditional distribution. All told then we take $X \sim N(\mu, \sigma^2)$ and $(X^*|X,Y) \sim N(X, \tau^2\sigma^2)$ as a simple, prototypical measurement error scenario. Note that with the chosen parameterization $\tau = SD(X^*|X)/SD(X)$ can be interpreted as the magnitude of the measurement error expressed as a fraction of the variability in the predictor X itself. For instance, $\tau = 0.1$ can be viewed as yielding 10% imprecision in the measurement of X.

Under the stated assumptions, standard distributional theory implies that (X, X^*) has a bivariate normal distribution. Using first the nondifferential property and then properties of this bivariate normal distribution, it follows that

$$
\begin{aligned}
E(Y|X^*) &= E\{E(Y|X)|X^*\} \\
&= \beta_0 + \beta_1 E(X|X^*) \\
&= \beta_0^* + \beta_1^* X_1^*,
\end{aligned}
$$

where

$$
\begin{aligned}
\beta_0^* - \beta_0 &= \frac{\mu\beta_1}{1 + \tau^2}, \\
\frac{\beta_1^*}{\beta_1} &= \frac{1}{1 + \tau^2}.
\end{aligned}
\tag{2.1}
$$

Thus the ordinary slope coefficient from a linear regression applied to sampled values of Y and X^* is an unbiased estimator of β_1^*. However, if this estimator is regarded as describing the relationship between Y and X, then a bias obtains—one is trying to estimate β_1 but actually estimating β_1^*. It is clear from (2.1) that β_1^* lies between zero and β_1. That is, in accord with the plots and simulations in Chapter 1, the effect of measurement error on the slope estimate is one of attenuation. As terminology we refer to (2.1) as the _attenuation factor (AF)_, while the magnitude of the _relative bias_ is $|(\beta_1^* - \beta_1)/\beta_1| = 1 - AF$. The basic relationship (2.1) between the magnitude of the mismeasurement and the extent of the attenuation is very well known, to the point that it is hard to trace an original reference. Fuller (1987) traces the literature as far back as Adcock (1877, 1878). Other historical references include Durbin (1954), and Cochran (1968).

In Figure 2.1 we plot the attenuation factor (2.1) as a function of τ, refer-

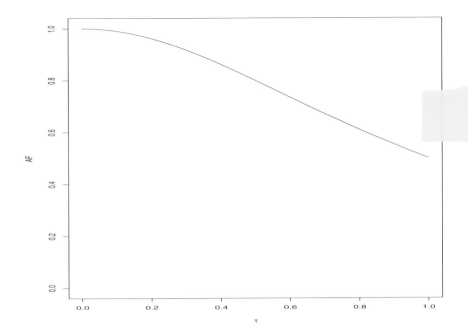

Figure 2.1 *Attenuation curve for linear regression with a single predictor. The curve is the attenuation factor* $(1 + \tau^2)^{-1}$ *plotted as a function of* τ.

ring to this as an *attenuation curve.* The first impression from the curve is that a moderate amount of measurement error does *not* cause a substantial attenuation. For instance, $\tau = 0.1$, interpreted as 10% measurement error, yields $AF = 0.99$, interpreted as a negligible 1% relative bias. Further along these lines, a 5% relative bias does not occur until we have 23% measurement error, and 33% measurement error is necessary to produce a 10% relative bias. It is reasonable to surmise that in this scenario one need not worry about the impact of measurement error unless this error is quite large. Of course, as discussed in Chapter 1, large measurement errors are quite common in epidemiological investigations. Moreover, we shall encounter plausible circumstances under which moderate measurement error causes much more severe bias.

2.2 More General Impact

Of course the expression (2.1) for the multiplicative bias induced by measurement error was derived under very specific assumptions about the distributions of X, $X^*|X$, and $Y|X, X^*$. It turns out, however, that a similar expression can be obtained in a much more general framework. In the absence of these distributional assumptions, the large-sample limit of estimated coefficients for regression of the response on the imprecise predictor can be compared to the corresponding limit for regression of the response on the precise predictor. To be more precise, by large-sample limit we mean the large-n limit of estimated coefficients from n independent and identically distributed realizations of the variables under consideration. We also expand the scope by considering a second predictor Z, which is precisely measured, to reflect the reality that most practical problems involve multiple regressors.

Before presenting the main result of this section we comment that by looking at large-sample limits our findings can be regarded as applying to different methods of parameter estimation. In particular, it is well known that in virtually any circumstance maximum likelihood and Bayesian estimators will tend to the same value as the sample size accumulates, regardless of whether the model leading to the estimators is correct or not. In fact throughout this chapter and the next our discussion of the impact of mismeasurement is not specific to the method of estimation. The Bayesian approach is introduced in Chapter 4 as a route to modelling and inference when the desire is to adjust for mismeasurement.

The impact of measurement error in linear regression with an additional precisely measured explanatory variable can be summarized as follows.

Result 2.1 *Assume that (Y, X, Z) jointly have finite second moments, and say X^* and (Z, Y) are conditionally independent given X, with $E(X^*|X) = X$ and $Var(X^*|X) = \tau^2 Var(X)$. Let β and β^* be the large-sample limiting coefficients from least-squares regression of Y on $(1, X, Z)$ and Y on $(1, X^*, Z)$ respectively. Then,*

$$\beta_0^* - \beta_0 = \beta_1 \left(\frac{\tau^2}{1 - \rho^2 + \tau^2} \right) \left\{ \mu_x - \rho \left(\frac{\sigma_x}{\sigma_z} \right) \mu_z \right\}, \qquad (2.2)$$

$$\frac{\beta_1^*}{\beta_1} = \frac{1}{1 + \tau^2/(1 - \rho^2)}, \qquad (2.3)$$

$$\beta_2^* - \beta_2 = \beta_1 \rho \left(\frac{\sigma_x}{\sigma_z} \right) \left(\frac{\tau^2}{1 - \rho^2 + \tau^2} \right), \quad \text{zero if } \rho = 0 \qquad (2.4)$$

where $\mu_x = E(X)$, $\mu_z = E(Z)$, $\sigma_x^2 = Var(X)$, $\sigma_z^2 = Var(Z)$, and $\rho = Cor(X, Z)$.

We do not offer a proof of Result 2.1 here. Rather, a somewhat more general result is proved later in Section 2.9. To be clear about the generality inherent in Result 2.1, note there is only reference to moments of (X, Z) and $X^*|X$, and in particular no normal distributions or other particular forms are imposed. Also, the expressions for β^* in terms of β make no reference to the actual distribution of the response Y given the precise predictors X and Z. While β describes the large-sample result of fitting a linear model for Y in terms of X and Z, there are no assumptions about the appropriateness of this model. Whereas expressions of the form (2.2) through (2.4) are very well known (see, for instance, Carroll, Ruppert and Stefanski, 1995), they are usually obtained under the assumption that Y really is related to (X, Z) according to the postulated linear model. The more general view of considering the relationship between the two sets of limiting coefficients is stressed in Gustafson and Le (2002). It is curious that at least asymptotically the bias induced by measurement error is unaffected by how well or poorly the postulated model for $Y|X,Z$ captures the actual relationship. Of course the generality of Result 2.1 does come at the price of being a statement about large-sample limits rather than finite-sample bias as in the previous section. We return to this point in Section 2.5.

Focussing on inference about the effect of X on Y, clearly the attenuation factor (2.3) generalizes (2.1) from the previous section, as the former reduces to the latter in the absence of correlation between X and Z. That is, the measurement error bias is unaffected by the inclusion of an additional precisely measured predictor Z only if this predictor is not correlated with X. On the other hand, the attenuating effect of measurement error worsens if Z is correlated with X. Note in particular that (2.3) goes to zero as ρ goes to one, indicating that very high correlation between X and Z yields extreme attenuation if the estimated effect of X^* is interpreted as estimating the effect of X.

To consider the role of correlation between X and Z more closely, Figure 2.2 displays attenuation curves, that is (2.3) as a function of τ, for various values of ρ. The display underscores that point that for moderate correlation the attenuation (2.3) is not much worse than (2.1) in the single predictor scenario. For large correlations, however, the attenuation is considerably stronger. Thus in practice one should be aware that strong correlations between the imprecisely measured predictor and other precisely measured predictors can warn of moderate measurement errors producing a substantial bias.

The other notable feature of Result 2.1 is that the measurement error in X also biases inference about the effect of Z on Y, despite the fact that Z is measured precisely. Furthermore, the bias $\beta_2^* - \beta_2$ scales with β_1 rather than with β_2. Whereas $\beta_1 = 0$ implies $\beta_1^* = 0$, so that one will not be misled about the absence of an effect of X on Y, $\beta_2 = 0$ will generally yield a nonzero value of β_2^*, provided both ρ and β_1 are nonzero. Thus an additional troubling aspect of measurement error is its ability to induce 'apparent significance' in other precisely measured predictors which actually have no effect on the response.

To further explore the impact of measurement error in X on inference about the effect of Z on Y, consider the situation where in fact Z is the explanatory variable of interest, but X is a suspected confounder. That is, the explanatory variable of interest can be measured precisely, but the confounding variable is subject to measurement error. It is easy to verify that if Y is regressed on $(1, Z)$ only then the large-sample limiting coefficient for Z will be

$$\tilde{\beta}_2 \;=\; \beta_2 + \rho \left(\frac{\sigma_x}{\sigma_z} \right) \beta_1,$$

where (β_1, β_2) are limiting coefficients as defined in Result 2.1. That is, if one really wants to estimate the impact of Z on Y given X, but X is omitted from the regression model, then one will be estimating $\tilde{\beta}_2$ rather than β_2 as desired.

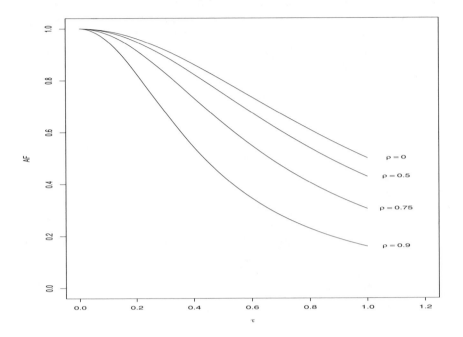

Figure 2.2 *Attenuation curves for linear regression with an additional precisely measured predictor. Each curve is (2.1) as a function of τ, with curves for $\rho = 0$, $\rho = 0.5$, $\rho = 0.75$, and $\rho = 0.9$ appearing.*

In this framework it is interesting to note that (2.4) can be re-expressed as

$$\beta_2^* = \{1 - w(\tau^2, \rho^2)\}\beta_2 + w(\tau^2, \rho^2)\tilde{\beta}_2, \qquad (2.5)$$

where

$$w(\tau^2, \rho^2) = \frac{1}{1 + (1 - \rho^2)/\tau^2}.$$

Thus the limiting coefficient for Z is a weighted combination of β_2, which is completely adjusted for confounding, and $\tilde{\beta}_2$, which is completely unadjusted for confounding. When $\tau = 0$ (or $\rho = 0$) all the weight is on the adjusted coefficient, but as τ goes to infinity (or ρ goes to one) all the weight goes to the unadjusted coefficient. In this sense measurement error in a confounder leads to some loss in the ability to control for the confounder in the analysis. This point is made in the case of categorical explanatory variables by Greenland (1980). We also note that correlation between X and Z imparts a 'double-whammy' in that a larger ρ corresponds to a bigger discrepancy between β_2 and $\tilde{\beta}_2$, as well as more weight on $\tilde{\beta}_2$ in (2.5).

Of course Result 2.1 is still limiting in that only one additional precise predictor is considered. Many practical problems will involve numerous such pre-

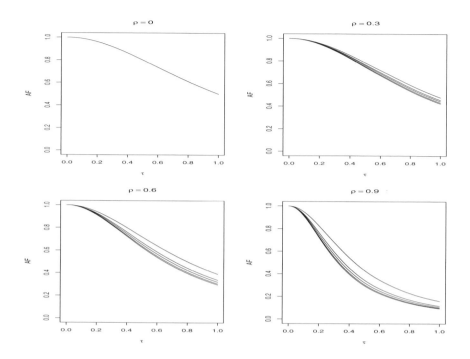

Figure 2.3 *Attenuation curves for linear regression with multiple equi-correlated pre-dictors. Each panel corresponds to a different value of the common correlation ρ. Each curve is the attenuation factor (2.21) as a function of τ. The curves are point-wise decreasing in d, the number of additional precise predictors included in the regression. Curves for $d = 1$, $d = 3$, $d = 5$, $d = 10$, and $d = 20$ appear.*

dictors. Later in Section 2.9 we state and prove Result 2.6 which handles any number of additional precise predictors. The resulting expressions are more unwieldy, but one easily-studied scenario involves equi-correlated predictors. That is, say that X^* and d precise predictors $Z_1, \ldots, Z_d$ are measured, with $\rho = Cor(X, Z_i) = Cor(Z_i, Z_j)$ for all i and j. The expression (2.21) in Section 2.9 gives the attenuation factor in this scenario. Plots of the attenuation curve for various values of d and ρ appear in Figure 2.3. For $\rho > 0$ the attenuation is seen to worsen as the number of additional predictors d increases, but this effect is fairly slight. Thus in practice the presence of many additional pre-cise predictors is only a mild indication of more severe attenuation due to measurement error.

2.3 Multiplicative Measurement Error

In the previous section the imprecision in the predictor arose from *additive* measurement error. We now turn to the case of *multiplicative* measurement error. That is, we consider situations where the amount of imprecision in the measurement of a positive predictor is proportional to the actual value of the predictor. Many predictors in biostatistical and epidemiological settings are subject to this sort of measurement error.

A first thought is that multiplicative measurement error can be converted to additive measurement error simply by transforming the predictor in question to the logarithmic scale. Indeed, say that U is the positive explanatory variable and U^* is its imprecise surrogate. We might define the measurement error as being multiplicative if the conditional distribution of U^*/U given U does not depend on U. This is equivalent to saying that the conditional distribution of $X^* - X$ does not depend on X, where $X = \log U$ and $X^* = \log U^*$, which might similarly be thought of as a characterization of additive measurement error. Consequently, separate treatments of additive and multiplicative measurement error are not really required. What is needed, however, is consideration of which function of X (or equivalently which function of U) is used as a regressor in the linear model for the response variable.

Consider the scenario where the positive predictor U and an additional predictor Z are the explanatory variables of interest, but a surrogate U^* and Z are observed. The investigator must postulate a model for Y in term of U and Z. If he chooses $\log U$ and Z as regressors but instead actually uses $\log U^*$ and Z, then Result 2.1 applies. On the other hand, if U itself or perhaps some power of U is used as a regressor then Result 2.1 is not applicable. The next result deals with these possibilities. For consistency with Result 2.1 it is expressed in terms of X^* arising from X via additive measurement error, but as discussed it can be viewed as dealing with $U^* = \exp(X^*)$ arising from $U = \exp(X)$ via multiplicative measurement error. The framework of the result and the attenuation factor determined are somewhat similar to work of Lyles and Kupper (1997), who go on to consider adjustments for mismeasurement in this context. More generally, though, there is little literature concerned with situations where the scale on which the mismeasured predictor is subject to additive measurement error differs from the scale on which the predictor appears in the outcome model.

Result 2.2 *Assume that (Y, e^{kX}, Z) jointly have finite second moments. Say X^* and (Z, Y) are conditionally independent given X. Let $\sigma^2 = Var(X)$ and assume $X^*|X \sim N(X, \tau^2\sigma^2)$. Let β be the large-sample limiting coefficients from linear regression of Y on $(1, e^{kX}, Z)$, and let β^* be the large-sample limiting coefficients from linear regression of Y on $(1, e^{kX^*}, Z)$. Then*

$$\frac{\beta_1^*}{\beta_1} = \frac{1}{\exp(k^2\sigma^2\tau^2/2)\left[1 + c\left\{\exp(k^2\sigma^2\tau^2) - 1\right\}\right]}, \qquad (2.6)$$

where

$$c = \frac{E\left(e^{2kX}\right)}{Var\left(e^{kX}\right)\left\{1 - Cor\left(e^{kX}, Z\right)^2\right\}}. \qquad (2.7)$$

A proof of this result is deferred to Section 2.9.

In examining (2.6), clearly the denominator is greater than one and increasing in τ, so again an attenuating bias results from the measurement error. Moreover, from (2.7) the attenuation is seen to worsen with increasing correlation between the precise regressors $\exp(kX)$ and Z. Note that the conditions in Result 2.2 are a little more restrictive than those in Result 2.1. In particular, normality of $X^*|X$ is now required to obtain somewhat tractable expressions.

It is somewhat instructive to consider a Taylor series approximation to the denominator of (2.6), expanding in τ about zero. The first derivative term vanishes, giving the small τ approximation

$$\frac{\beta_1^*}{\beta_1} \approx \frac{1}{1 + (0.5 + c)k^2\sigma^2\tau^2}.$$

Of course this has a similar form to (2.3) in the situation where X itself is considered as the regressor.

To consider a specific case more clearly, say X and Z have a bivariate normal distribution, and let $\rho = Cor(X, Z)$. It is straightforward to verify that (2.7) specializes to

$$c = \frac{e^{k^2\sigma^2}}{\left(e^{k^2\sigma^2} - 1\right)\left[1 - \left\{k^2\sigma^2/\left(e^{k^2\sigma^2} - 1\right)\right\}\rho^2\right]}.$$

In this scenario $U = \exp(X)$ has a log-normal distribution, with $\sigma = SD(X)$ becoming a shape parameter which governs the skewness of this distribution. The top panels in Figure 2.4 display the log-normal density function for U when $\sigma = 0.25$, $\sigma = 1$, and $\sigma = 1.75$. In each case $\mu = E(X) = 0$ so that the median of U is one. Note, however, that this simply fixes the scale of U, and the bias (2.6) will not depend on μ. The panels below each density give multiplicative bias curves when σ takes the value in question, for three different values of $\rho = Cor(X, Z)$. Specifically, three curves appear in each panel. The solid curve is (2.6) with $k = 1$, describing a situation where U itself is used as a regressor. The dashed curve is (2.6) with $k = 0.5$, describing a situation where $U^{1/2}$ is used as a regressor. Finally, the dotted curve is (2.3) from Result 2.1, describing the situation where $\log U$ is used as a regressor.

The figure shows that when $\sigma = 0.25$ the density of U is quite symmetric, and for each value of ρ the three bias curves corresponding to the three choices of regressor are nearly indistinguishable. When $\sigma = 1$, however, the density of U is quite skewed, with a long right tail. In this case, unless ρ is very large, there are substantial differences between the biases for the three choices of regressor. Specifically, the use of U itself leads to the most attenuation, followed by the use of $U^{1/2}$ and then the use of $\log U$. These differences are magnified when $\sigma = 1.75$, corresponding to even more skewness in the distribution of U. Again, however, the behaviour when $\rho = 0.9$ is not in accord with the behaviour for $\rho = 0$ and $\rho = 0.5$.

We surmise that multiplicative measurement error has the potential to yield particularly strong attenuation in the estimated regression coefficient for the regressor subject to measurement error. Specifically, this potential is realized if (i) the positive explanatory variable subject to multiplicative measurement error has a skewed distribution, and (ii) this variable itself, or possibly a power transformation of this variable, enters the outcome model linearly. On the other hand, if the regressor is obtained via a log transformation, then the induced bias reduces to that obtained in the additive error case as described in Result 2.1. Of course this finding makes good intuitive sense. If U itself is used as a regressor and its distribution has a long right tail, then the multiplicative measurement error yields the largest errors for a few potentially influential data points in the tail of the distribution.

2.4 Multiple Mismeasured Predictors

Of course more than one of the predictors in a given problem may be subject to measurement error. The following result describes what happens when both explanatory variables under consideration are subject to additive measurement error. In addition to allowing for correlation between the two precise predictors, we allow for correlation between the two additive errors. Such dependence would be plausible in a number of circumstances. For instance, if the two regressors are daily levels of two ambient pollutants, it is plausible that the instrumentation used to measure these levels could yield correlated errors in the two measurements.

Result 2.3 *Assume (Y, X_1, X_2) jointly have finite second moments, where each X_i has been scaled so that $E(X_i) = 0$ and $Var(X_i) = 1$. Let $\rho = Cor(X_1, X_2)$. Assume $X^* = (X_1^*, X_2^*)$ is conditionally independent of Y given $X = (X_1, X_2)$, with $E(X_i^*|X) = X_i$ and*

$$Var(X^*|X) = \begin{pmatrix} \tau_1^2 & \lambda\tau_1\tau_2 \\ \lambda\tau_1\tau_2 & \tau_2^2 \end{pmatrix}.$$

Let $\beta = (\beta_0, \beta_1, \beta_2)'$ be the large-sample limiting coefficients from linear regression of Y on $(1, X_1, X_2)'$, and let $\beta^* = (\beta_0^*, \beta_1^*, \beta_2^*)'$ be the large-sample limiting coefficients from linear regression of Y on $(1, X_1^*, X_2^*)'$. Then

$$\beta_1^* = \frac{(1 + \tau_2^2 - \rho^2 - \rho\lambda\tau_1\tau_2)\beta_1 + (\rho\tau_2^2 - \lambda\tau_1\tau_2)\beta_2}{(1 + \tau_1^2)(1 + \tau_2^2) - (\rho + \lambda\tau_1\tau_2)^2}, \qquad (2.8)$$

with a symmetric expression obtaining for β_2^*.

A proof of Result 2.3 is not given, but can be established along the same lines as the proof Result 2.6 in Section 2.9. Such expressions are well established in the literature (see, for example, Carroll, Ruppert and Stefanski 1995, Sec. 2.2.4), but again they are typically derived under the assumption that the postulated linear model for Y given (X_1, X_2) is correct. Thus we emphasize that again in this scenario the bias induced by measurement error does not depend on the actual distribution of the response given the precise predictors.

With variances τ_1^2 and τ_2^2 and correlations ρ and λ at play, it is difficult to glean much understanding by examining (2.8) directly. Rather, we fix $(\beta_1, \beta_2) = (0.5, 0.25)$, and compute (β_1^*, β_2^*) for various values of τ_1, τ_2, ρ, and λ. The results appear in Table 2.1.

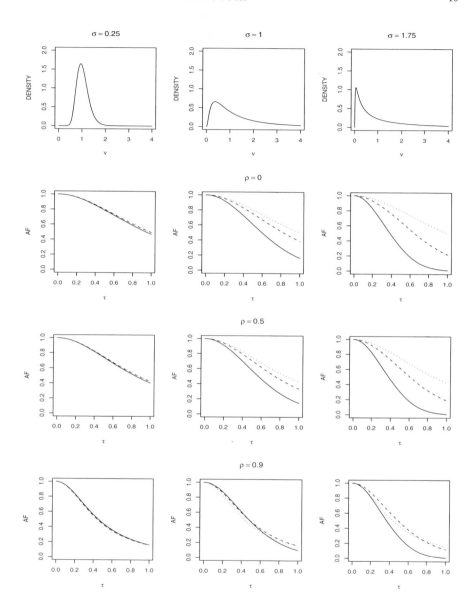

Figure 2.4 *Log-normal densities and corresponding attenuation curves. The columns of plots correspond to log-normal shape parameters $\sigma = 0.25$, $\sigma = 1$, and $\sigma = 1.75$. The top panels give the log-normal density functions scaled to have median zero. The panels below give the resulting attenuation curves, with the three rows corresponding to different values of $\rho = Cor(\log U, Z)$. Each panel contains three curves. The solid curve corresponds to the use of U as a regressor, the dashed curve corresponds to the use of $U^{1/2}$ as a regressor, and the dotted curve corresponds to the use of $\log U$ as a regressor.*

λ	τ_1	τ_2	$\rho = 0.0$	$\rho = 0.5$	$\rho = 0.9$
0.0	0.2	0.2	(0.48 , 0.24)	(0.48 , 0.25)	(0.46 , 0.28)
	0.2	0.5	(0.48 , 0.20)	(0.51 , 0.20)	(0.56 , 0.15)
	0.5	0.2	(0.40 , 0.24)	(0.38 , 0.30)	(0.25 , 0.45)
	0.5	0.5	(0.40 , 0.20)	(0.40 , 0.24)	(0.37 , 0.30)
0.5	0.2	0.2	(0.48 , 0.23)	(0.48 , 0.24)	(0.47 , 0.26)
	0.2	0.5	(0.47 , 0.18)	(0.51 , 0.18)	(0.61 , 0.10)
	0.5	0.2	(0.39 , 0.22)	(0.38 , 0.28)	(0.22 , 0.47)
	0.5	0.5	(0.38 , 0.16)	(0.40 , 0.20)	(0.37 , 0.26)
0.9	0.2	0.2	(0.47 , 0.22)	(0.48 , 0.23)	(0.48 , 0.24)
	0.2	0.5	(0.47 , 0.17)	(0.51 , 0.16)	(0.67 , 0.03)
	0.5	0.2	(0.39 , 0.21)	(0.37 , 0.27)	(0.19 , 0.49)
	0.5	0.5	(0.38 , 0.13)	(0.40 , 0.17)	(0.40 , 0.20)

Table 2.1 *Values of (β_1^*, β_2^*) when both predictors are subject to additive measurement error. The limiting coefficients in the absence of measurement error are $(\beta_1, \beta_2) = (0.5, 0.25)$. Various values of $\tau_i = Var(X_i^*|X)$, $\rho = Cor(X_1, X_2)$, and $\lambda = Cor(X_1^*, X_2^*|X)$ are considered.*

Perhaps the most notable observation from Table 2.1 is that the effect of imprecision in two explanatory variables is not always attenuation. That is, some scenarios yield $|\beta_1^*| > |\beta_1|$, or $|\beta_2^*| > |\beta_2|$. Also, the relative magnitudes of the estimated effects can be distorted by the measurement error, as $\beta_1^* < \beta_2^*$ in some scenarios even though $\beta_1 = 2\beta_2$. In short, with more than one imprecise covariate there is more danger of drawing substantively erroneous conclusions, and the nature of the induced bias is not easily predicted without knowledge of the magnitudes of the measurement errors, the correlation between the underlying precise predictors, and the correlation between the measurement errors.

Given that Result 2.3 applies after each regressor has been standardized, we can regard the predictor with the larger $|\beta_i|$ as being the more important of the two in explaining variation in Y. Of course if the data are analyzed without considering the measurement error then the predictor with the larger $|\beta_i^*|$ will be *apparently* more important. We have already noted from Table 2.1 that the predictor which is apparently more important may not be actually more important. Obviously this sort of *reversal* is very damaging, as it leads to a qualitatively wrong assessment of the relationship between the response and the predictors.

Looking more closely at Table 2.1, we see reversals when the two underlying precise predictors are highly correlated, but the one that is actually more important is measured with more error than the other. To study the potential for reversal more carefully, consider the case of uncorrelated measurement errors, that is $\lambda = 0$. Say $\beta_1 > 0$ and $\beta_2 > 0$, with $\beta_1/\beta_2 = \gamma > 1$. From (2.8) one would mistakenly conclude that X_2 is more important if

$$(1 + \rho\gamma)\tau_1^2 + (1 - \rho^2) \quad > \quad (\gamma + \rho)\tau_2^2 + \gamma(1 - \rho^2). \qquad (2.9)$$

If the precise predictors have little or no correlation, then reversal is not likely to be a problem. For instance, say $\gamma = 1.25$, $\tau_2 = 0.1$, and $\rho = 0$. Then (2.9) shows that reversal would require a substantial measurement error of $\tau_1 > 0.51$. The situation changes, however, when the precise predictors are highly correlated. In fact, as ρ tends to one, the inequality (2.9) tends to $\tau_1 > \tau_2$, for any value of γ. That is, in the limit of perfect correlation the more precisely measured predictor will be implicated as the more important predictor, regardless of the actual underlying relationship between Y and X. As examples with strong but not perfect correlation, again say that $\gamma = 1.25$ and $\tau_2 = 0.1$. When $\rho = 0.75$, (2.9) shows that $\tau_1 > 0.26$ is required for reversal, and when $\rho = 0.9$, $\tau_1 > 0.18$ is required. Thus reversal is clearly more of a danger if the two predictors in question are highly correlated. Related questions of whether the right explanatory variable is implicated in an environmetrics scenario are considered by Zidek, Wong, Le and Burnett (1996).

2.5 What about Variability and Small Samples?

So far in this chapter we have used large-sample limits to compare regression coefficients based on imprecise predictors to those based on precise predictors. An obvious question is how well do the resulting asymptotic biases reflect what actually happens for a particular fixed sample size.

To investigate we return to the context of Section 2.2 and perform a simulation study with three different distributions for the precise predictors (X, Z) and two different distributions for the response Y given these predictors. Thus six scenarios are considered in all. The three different distributions for the predictors all have $E(X) = E(Z) = 0$, $Var(X) = Var(Z) = 1$, and $\rho = Cor(X, Z) = 2/3$. Thus by Result 2.1 the large-sample multiplicative bias in estimating the effect of X is the same in all six scenarios.

To be more specific, the first distribution of predictors is 'short-tailed.' Both X and Z are taken to have uniform distributions on $(-\sqrt{3}, \sqrt{3})$. But rather than having a jointly uniform distribution, some probability is moved from the quadrants where X and Z have differing signs to the quadrants where X and Z have the same signs, to achieve $Cor(X, Z) = 2/3$. The second distribution of predictors is simply bivariate normal. The third distribution is bivariate Student's t, with four degrees of freedom for each component and the desired covariance matrix.

Both distributions for the response involve a normal distribution for $Y|X, Z$ with $Var(Y|X, Z) = 1$. In the first case,

$$E(Y|X, Z) = X + (0.5)Z, \qquad (2.10)$$

giving scenarios in which the postulated linear model for the response given the precise predictors is correct. In the second case,

$$E(Y|X, Z) = e^X + (0.5)I\{Z > 0\}, \qquad (2.11)$$

under which the postulated linear model is clearly not correct. Result 2.1 indicates that asymptotically the measurement error bias is the same for all distributions of the response given the precise predictors, but by trying both (2.10) and (2.11) we will see how well this translates to fixed sample sizes.

We simulate 2000 samples of (Y, X, Z, X^*) for each scenario and for each of three sample sizes: $n = 50$, $n = 200$, and $n = 400$. In each instance the measurement error is induced via $X^*|X, Z, Y \sim N(X, \tau^2)$ with $\tau = 0.5$. For each sample we compute $\hat{\beta}$, the estimated coefficients from regression of Y on $(1, X, Z)$, and $\hat{\beta}^*$, the estimated coefficients from regression of Y on $(1, X^*, Z)$. Figure 2.5 uses boxplots to illustrate the sampling distribution of the finite sample *realized attenuation*, $\hat{\beta}_1^*/\hat{\beta}_1$, for each scenario and sample size. The large-sample attenuation factor (2.3), which equals $20/29$ in the present scenario, is also marked on the plots.

The Figure indicates considerable variability in the sampling distribution of the realized attenuation, especially when n is small. Even when $n = 50$, however, the large-sample attenuation factor is a very good descriptor of the centre of the sampling distribution. In particular, the centre exhibits very little variation across scenarios. The same is not true of the spread in the sampling distributions. Somewhat predictably, the realized attenuation is more variable when (X, Z) have the long-tailed distribution, especially when the response variable is not linear in the predictors. For the other (X, Z) distributions, however, the distribution of the realized attenuation is almost the same for the two response distributions. In all, the simulations lend credence to the large-sample attenuation factor as a good descriptor of the measurement error impact in smaller samples.

Another point concerning the variability of naive estimators which don't correct for measurement error concerns the reported uncertainty associated with such estimators. To make the point simply, consider the scenario above where the distribution of X is normal and (2.10) holds, so that $E(Y|X, Z)$ and $E(Y|X^*, Z)$ are both linear in their arguments, with coefficient vectors β and β^* respectively. Naive estimation ignoring measurement error yields $\hat{\beta}_1^* \pm 1.96 \times SE[\hat{\beta}_1^*]$ as a reported 95% confidence interval for β_1. Of course the primary problem here is that the interval is centred in the wrong place, as has been discussed. However, there is also the secondary problem that the interval is too narrow. Intuitively, it does not reflect the loss of information associated with measuring only X^* and not X. To elaborate, say the attenuation factor is known to be $AF \in (0, 1)$, i.e., $\beta_1^* = AF\beta_1$. Then a simple corrected estimate for β_1 would be $AF^{-1}\hat{\beta}_1^*$. Clearly an approximate 95% confidence interval centred at this estimate must take the form $AF^{-1}\hat{\beta}_1^* \pm 1.96 \times AF^{-1}SE[\hat{\beta}_1^*]$, in order to achieve the nominal coverage. This arises easily by transforming the approximate confidence interval for β_1^*. Thus to construct an appropriate interval estimate from the naive interval we must both move the centre of the interval *and* make the interval wider by a factor of AF^{-1}. While this chapter and the next emphasize the bias inherent in naive estimation, it should be remembered that underestimation of apparent variability is also manifested.

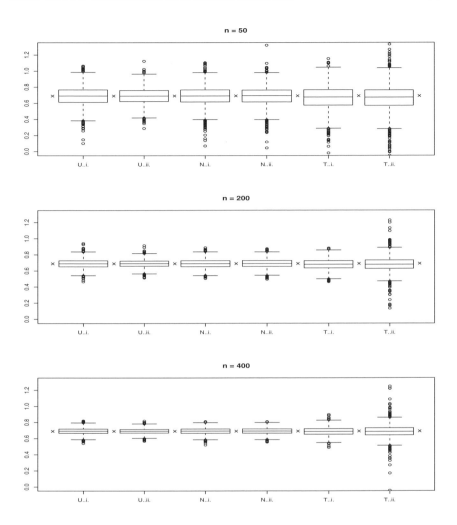

Figure 2.5 *Sampling distribution of the realized attenuation for six scenarios and three sample sizes. At each sample size the first two boxplots correspond to the modified uniform distribution of predictors, the second two correspond to the bivariate normal distribution, and the last two correspond to the bivariate t distribution with four degrees of freedom. In each pair, the first boxplot corresponds to the linear response (2.10) and the second to the nonlinear response (2.11). The crosses between the boxplots mark the asymptotic bias which is the same for all scenarios. Each boxplot is based on* 2000 *simulated samples.*

2.6 Logistic Regression

Up to this point we have considered the bias induced by measurement error when linear regression is used to relate a continuous response variable to explanatory variables. Of course many analyses that arise in biostatistics and epidemiology in particular involve a binary response variable. In such cases the most common inferential procedure is logistic regression, which is one particular case of a generalized linear model. Roughly stated, a 'folk theorem' pervading statistics is that generalized linear models behave very similarly to linear models. We put this to the test by examining the impact of measurement error when logistic regression is applied to data with a binary outcome variable. There is a considerable literature on measurement error in binary regression models, though some of this focusses on probit regression rather than logistic regression for the sake of numerical tractability (Carroll, Spiegelman, Lan, Bailey and Abbott, 1984).

Unfortunately, closed-form expressions for the bias induced by measurement error in logistic regression do not exist. Thus some numerical work is required to mimic analytic findings such as Results 2.1, 2.2, and 2.3 for linear regression. For instance, consider the following scenario which parallels that of Result 2.1. An investigator is interested in a logistic regression of a binary outcome variable Y on continuous regressors X and Z. Due to measurement error, however, he actually performs a logistic regression of Y on X^* and Z, where X^* and (Y, Z) are conditionally independent given X, $E(X^*|X) = X$, and $Var(X^*|X) = \tau^2 Var(X)$. If we define $T = (1, X, Z)'$ and let β be the large-sample limiting coefficients from logistic regression of Y on the components of T, then standard large-sample theory (e.g., White 1980) for logistic regression gives β as the solution to a system of three equations, compactly denoted in vector form as

$$E\left[T\left\{Y - \frac{1}{1 + \exp(-\beta'T)}\right\}\right] = 0. \qquad (2.12)$$

Similarly, if $T^* = (1, X^*, Z)'$ and β^* is the large-sample limiting coefficients from logistic regression of Y on T^*, then

$$E\left[T^*\left\{Y - \frac{1}{1 + \exp(-\beta^{*\prime}T^*)}\right\}\right] = 0. \qquad (2.13)$$

Stefanski and Carroll (1985) use a variant of (2.13) to provide large-sample approximations to the bias incurred in estimating β_1 when using T^* rather than T as regressors.

We proceed by noting that under the stated conditions $E(X^*Y) = E(XY)$, and hence $E(T^*Y) = E(TY)$. This leads to β^* as a function of β being determined as the solution to

$$E\left[T^*\left\{\frac{1}{1 + \exp(-\beta^{*\prime}T^*)}\right\}\right] = E\left[T\left\{\frac{1}{1 + \exp(-\beta'T)}\right\}\right]. \qquad (2.14)$$

While the system of equations (2.14) does not have an analytic solution, its form implies that the relationship between β^* and β is not affected by

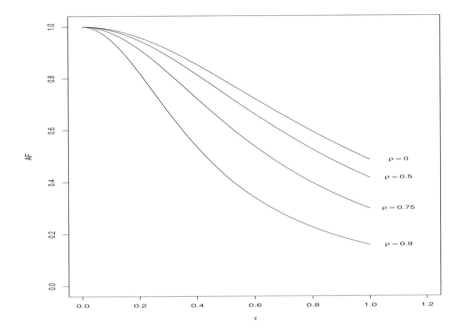

Figure 2.6 *Attenuation curves for logistic regression in the case of one additional precise predictor. Each curve is β_1^*/β_1 as a function of τ, with curves for $\rho = 0$, $\rho = 0.5$, $\rho = 0.75$, and $\rho = 0.9$ appearing. The large-sample limiting coefficients for logistic regression of Y on X and Z are taken to be $\beta = (0, 0.5, 0.25)'$.*

the actual distribution of $Y|X, Z$. This is in accord with the linear regression case as per Result 2.1. On the other hand, some nice features of the earlier result do not carry over to the present setting. For instance, in Result 2.1 the attenuation factor β_1^*/β_1 is the same for all values of β. The solution to (2.14) does not have this property, although our numerical experience suggests that the dependence of β_1^*/β_1 on β is quite mild.

In Section 2.9 we state and prove Result 2.7 which yields a variant of (2.14), and describe a computational scheme to compute β^* for a given β approximately. In particular, this scheme uses a combination of Monte Carlo simulation and the solution of 'pseudo' logistic regression likelihood equations. This scheme is applied to solve (2.14) in a scenario where X and Z have a bivariate normal distribution with standardized marginals, $X^*|X$ is normally distributed, and $\beta = (0, 0.5, 0.25)'$. Attenuation curves, that is β_1^*/β_1 as a function of τ, appear in Figure 2.6, for various values of $\rho = Cor(X, Z)$. These curves bear a very strong resemblance to those for linear regression in Figure 2.2. This supports the notion that the impact of measurement error in logistic regression is very similar to the impact in linear regression.

We also investigate the effects of multiplicative measurement error in logistic regression, along the lines of Result 2.2 and the ensuing discussion in Section 2.3. Say (X, Z) have a bivariate normal distribution with $E(X) = E(Z) = 0$, $Var(X) = \sigma^2$, and $Var(Z) = 1$, while $X^*|X, Z, Y \sim N(X, \tau^2\sigma^2)$. In analogy to Result 2.2 we consider logistic regression of Y on regressors $T^* = (1, e^{kX^*}, Z)'$ in lieu of $T = (1, e^{kX}, Z)'$. Again Result 2.7 and the associated computational scheme permit approximation of the large-sample coefficients β^* for T^* given large-sample coefficients β for T.

To illustrate we fix $\beta = (0, 0.5, 0.25)'$, and then compute attenuation curves which appear in Figure 2.7. As before, the additive measurement error for X can be regarded as multiplicative measurement error for $V = \exp(X)$. Three different values of $\sigma = Var(X)$ and three different values of $\rho = Cor(X, Z)$ are considered. In each case the solid curve corresponds to using $V^* = \exp(X^*)$ as a regressor in lieu of $V = \exp(X)$, the dashed curve corresponds to the use of $(V^*)^{1/2} = \exp(X^*/2)$ in lieu of $V^{1/2} = \exp(X/2)$, and the dotted curve corresponds to the use of $\log V^* = X^*$ in lieu of $\log V = X$. Thus Figure 2.7 describes the same scenarios as Figure 2.4, except that linear regression for a continuous response variable has been replaced with logistic regression for a binary response variable. The curves in the two figures are strikingly similar, again supporting the notion that the impact of measurement error in logistic regression mimics the impact in linear regression.

Finally we consider logistic regression with two regressors that are both subject to measurement error. Again the mathematical details are subsumed by Result 2.7 and the associated computational scheme. The joint distribution of $X = (X_1, X_2)$ and $X^* = (X_1^*, X_2^*)$ is taken to be multivariate normal, with moment structure exactly as in Result 2.3 for linear regression. In particular, X_1 and X_2 are both standardized, while $\tau_i^2 = Var(X_i^*|X)$, $\lambda = Cor(X_1^*, X_2^*|X)$, and $\rho = Cor(X_1, X_2)$. The large-sample limiting coefficients for logistic regression of Y on $(1, X_1, X_2)$ are taken to be $\beta = (0, 0.5, 0.25)'$. Table 2.2 gives (β_1^*, β_2^*) (the intercept β_0^* is not shown) under the same combinations of τ_i, ρ, and λ considered in Table 2.1 for linear regression. The agreement of the tables is very striking; entries differ by no more than 0.01 between the linear regression and logistic regression scenarios. Once again we have strong support for the notion that measurement error impacts logistic regression in very much the same manner that it impacts linear regression.

2.7 Beyond Nondifferential and Unbiased Measurement Error

To this point we have considered the impact of 'fair' measurement error, meaning (i) on some scale the imprecise predictor is an unbiased estimate of the precise predictor, and (ii) the distribution of the imprecise predictor given the precise predictor, other predictors and the response depends only on the precise predictor. However there are realistic situations where measurement error may be biased or differential. We briefly consider two such scenarios. Proofs of the results are omitted, as they are much in the spirit of the proof of Result 2.6 given in Section 2.9.

First, in the context of Result 2.1 we replace $E(X|X^*) = X$ with $E(X^*|X) =$

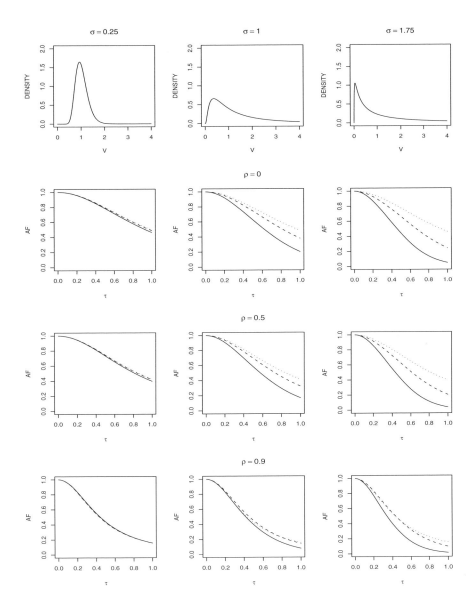

Figure 2.7 *Log normal densities and corresponding multiplicative bias curves for logistic regression with multiplicative measurement error. The top panels give density functions for $V = \exp(X)$, where $X \sim N(0, \sigma^2)$, for $\sigma = 0.25$, $\sigma = 1$, and $\sigma = 1.75$. The panels below give multiplicative bias curves for different values of $\rho = Cor(X, Z)$. Each panel contains three curves. The solid curve corresponds to the use of V as a regressor, the dashed curve corresponds to the use of $V^{1/2}$ as a regressor, and the dotted curve corresponds to the use of $\log V$ as a regressor. The large-sample limit for logistic regression of Y on $(1, V, Z)$ is taken to be $\beta = (0, 0.5, 0.25)$ in each case.*

λ	τ_1	τ_2	$\rho = 0.0$	$\rho = 0.5$	$\rho = 0.9$
0.0	0.2	0.2	(0.48 , 0.24)	(0.48 , 0.25)	(0.45 , 0.28)
	0.2	0.5	(0.48 , 0.20)	(0.50 , 0.20)	(0.56 , 0.15)
	0.5	0.2	(0.39 , 0.24)	(0.38 , 0.30)	(0.25 , 0.45)
	0.5	0.5	(0.39 , 0.20)	(0.40 , 0.24)	(0.36 , 0.29)
0.5	0.2	0.2	(0.47 , 0.23)	(0.48 , 0.24)	(0.46 , 0.26)
	0.2	0.5	(0.47 , 0.18)	(0.50 , 0.18)	(0.60 , 0.10)
	0.5	0.2	(0.38 , 0.22)	(0.37 , 0.28)	(0.22 , 0.47)
	0.5	0.5	(0.38 , 0.16)	(0.39 , 0.20)	(0.36 , 0.26)
0.9	0.2	0.2	(0.47 , 0.22)	(0.48 , 0.23)	(0.48 , 0.24)
	0.2	0.5	(0.46 , 0.16)	(0.51 , 0.16)	(0.66 , 0.03)
	0.5	0.2	(0.38 , 0.20)	(0.37 , 0.27)	(0.19 , 0.49)
	0.5	0.5	(0.37 , 0.13)	(0.39 , 0.16)	(0.39 , 0.20)

Table 2.2 *Values of* (β_1^*, β_2^*) *when both regressors in a logistic regression are subject to additive measurement error. The limiting coefficients in the absence of measurement error are* $(\beta_0, \beta_1, \beta_2) = (0, 0.5, 0.25)$. *Various values of* $\tau_i = Var(X_i^*|X_i)$, $\rho = Cor(X_1, X_2)$, *and* $\lambda = Cor(X_1^*, X_2^*|X)$ *are considered.*

$a + bX$. Thus we are considering a systematic bias in the measurement of the predictor. The modified result is as follows.

Result 2.4 *Assume that* (Y, X, Z) *jointly have finite second moments, where* X *and* Z *have been scaled so that* $E(X) = E(Z) = 0$ *and* $Var(X) = Var(Z) = 1$. *Say* X^* *and* (Z, Y) *are conditionally independent given* X, *with* $E(X^*|X) = a + bX$ *and* $Var(X^*|X) = \tau^2$. *Let* β *and* β^* *be the large-sample limiting coefficients from least-squares regression of* Y *on* $(1, X, Z)$ *and* Y *on* $(1, X^*, Z)$ *respectively. Then,*

$$\frac{\beta_1^*}{\beta_1} = \frac{1}{b + \tau^2/\{b(1 - \rho^2)\}}. \tag{2.15}$$

It is not surprising that the attenuation factor does not depend on a. Invariance considerations imply that translation error in the form of adding the same constant to each predictor will not have any effect on the estimate of a slope parameter. On the other hand, a multiplicative bias in the measurement process, as manifested when $b \neq 1$, does alter the multiplicative bias in the estimated coefficient. For moderate measurement error $(\tau^2 < 1 - \rho^2)$, (2.15) is a decreasing function of b in a neighbourhood of $b = 1$. Thus compared to the $b = 1$ case, attenuation is worse when the measurement error involves an upward bias $(b > 1)$ which tends to overstate the magnitude of the predictor.

There are also plausible situations under which the measurement error is differential. Say Y is an indicator of health status coded such that larger values correspond to poorer health, while X is the level of a possible risk factor. If X^* is ascertained by some sort of 'self-report' mechanism, there may be a possibility of differential measurement error. Depending on society's view of Y and X, individuals with high levels of Y might have a tendency to blame X

for their condition. Or perhaps individuals with high levels of Y might want to deny the possibility that X has caused their condition. In either scenario, differential measurement error can result. A modification of Result 2.1 which considers this possibility is as follows.

Result 2.5 *Assume that (Y, X, Z, X^*) jointly have finite second moments, where X and Z have been scaled so that $E(X) = E(Z) = 0$ and $Var(X) = Var(Z) = 1$. Say $E(X^*|X, Z) = X$ and $Var(X^*|X, Z) = \tau^2$, but X^* and Y are not necessarily conditionally independent given (X, Z). Let β and β^* be the large-sample limiting coefficients from least-squares regression of Y on $(1, X, Z)$ and Y on $(1, X^*, Z)$ respectively. Then,*

$$\beta_1^* = \frac{\beta_1}{1 + \tau^2/(1 - \rho^2)} + \frac{\Delta}{1 - \rho^2 + \tau^2}, \tag{2.16}$$

where $\Delta = E\{Cov(X^*, Y|X, Z)\}$.

Note, in particular, that the two terms in (2.16) can push β_1^* in opposite directions. Say β_1 is positive. The first term in (2.16) corresponds to the usual attenuation factor. However, if X^* and Y are positively dependent given (X, Z), then $\Delta > 0$ and the second term in (2.16) has an accentuating effect on β_1^*. Thus the combined effect could be one of either attenuation or accentuation. The practical warning is to look out for situations where the measurement error may be differential. In particular, the impact of differential error is harder to predict in advance than the impact of nondifferential error.

2.8 Summary

Having now determined the bias due to measurement error in a number of scenarios, we can give some qualitative guidance on when this bias is likely to be substantial. Of course the first consideration is the magnitude of the measurement error, though this alone does not usually suffice to determine the bias in the corresponding regression coefficient. The next consideration is whether the predictor subject to measurement error is highly correlated with other precisely measured predictors. If so, a strong attenuation in the regression coefficient can result. Another consideration is whether the measurement error is additive or multiplicative. There is more potential for substantive bias in the second case, though whether this potential is realized depends on the shape of the predictor's distribution, and on how the predictor is included in the regression model. We also examined imprecision in several predictors, and 'unfair' measurement error that is either biased or differential. In these situations the nature of the bias in the regression coefficients is more complicated, and attenuation will not necessarily result. Overall, this chapter aims to gives some intuition about when adjustment for measurement error will be sorely needed, and when it will make only a slight difference.

Some of the expressions for bias presented in this chapter are either identical or very similar to expressions in the literature. In particular the books of

Fuller (1987) and Carroll, Ruppert and Stefanski (1995) cover much of the same ground. Typically, however, the context surrounding the expressions is somewhat different. In particular, the approach of comparing the large-sample limiting coefficients with imprecise predictors to the corresponding limit with precise predictors does not seem to have been stressed previously, except recently in Gustafson and Le (2002).

2.9 Mathematical Details

2.9.1 A Generalization of Result 2.1

Result 2.6 *Suppose that (Y, X, Z) jointly have finite second moments, where Y and X are scalar, and Z is a vector with d components. Without loss of generality assume X and the components of Z have been scaled so that $E(X) = E(Z_i) = 0$ and $Var(X) = Var(Z_i) = 1$. Furthermore, say X^* and (Z, Y) are conditionally independent given X, with $E(X^*|X) = X$ and $Var(X^*|X) = \tau^2$. Let β and β^* be the large-sample limiting coefficients from least-squares regression of Y on $(1, X, Z)$ and Y on $(1, X^*, Z)$ respectively. Then*

$$\beta_0^* = \beta_0,$$

$$\frac{\beta_1^*}{\beta_1} = \left(\frac{1}{1+\tau^2}\right)\left\{1 - \left(\frac{\tau^2}{1+\tau^2}\right) r'\left(R - \frac{rr'}{1+\tau^2}\right)^{-1} r\right\}, \quad (2.17)$$

$$\beta_2^* - \beta_2 = \left(\frac{\beta_1\tau^2}{1+\tau^2}\right)\left(R - \frac{rr'}{1+\tau^2}\right)^{-1} r,$$

where $R = E(ZZ')$ and $r = E(ZX)$. The scaling of X and Z implies that R is the $d \times d$ correlation matrix of Z, while r is the $d \times 1$ vector of correlations between X and the components of Z.

Note that we have assumed X and Z are standardized in order to simplify the foregoing expressions. However, it is a simple matter to transform the expressions to describe the nonstandardized situation, as in Result 2.1 for instance.

Proof of Result 2.6. Define $T = (1, X, Z)'$, $T^* = (1, X^*, Z)'$, and $M = E(TT')$, $N = E(T^*T^{*\prime})$. Standard results for wrong-model asymptotics imply that β solves $M\beta = E(TY)$ while β^* solves $N\beta^* = E(T^*Y)$. But from the assumed properties of X^* we have $E(X^*Y) = E\{YE(X^*|X, Z, Y)\} = E(YX)$, so that $E(T^*Y) = E(TY)$, and hence $\beta^* = N^{-1}M\beta$. Partition M and N so that the on-diagonal blocks are 2×2 and $d \times d$, and note that $M_{22} = N_{22} = E(ZZ') = R$. Furthermore,

$$M_{12} = \begin{pmatrix} 0 & \cdots & 0 \\ r_1 & \cdots & r_d \end{pmatrix}, \quad (2.18)$$

and since $E(ZX^*) = E\{ZE(X^*|X, Z)\} = E(ZX)$, $N_{12} = M_{12}$. Finally, note that $M_{11} = I$, while

$$N_{11} = \begin{pmatrix} 1 & 0 \\ 0 & 1+\tau^2 \end{pmatrix}. \quad (2.19)$$

Using the standard expression for the inverse of a partitioned matrix (see, for instance, Gentle 1998, p. 61) gives

$$
N^{-1}M \;=\; \begin{pmatrix} N_{11}^{-1}(I + M_{12}Z^{-1}M_{21}N_{11}^{-1}) & -N_{11}^{-1}M_{12}Z^{-1} \\ -Z^{-1}M_{21}N_{11}^{-1} & Z^{-1} \end{pmatrix} \times \\ \begin{pmatrix} I & M_{12} \\ M_{21} & M_{22} \end{pmatrix},
$$

where $Z = M_{22} - M_{21}N_{11}^{-1}M_{12}$. Carrying out the blocked multiplication gives

$$
N^{-1}M \;=\; \begin{pmatrix} N_{11}^{-1}\{I + M_{12}Z^{-1}M_{21}(N_{11}^{-1} - I)\} & 0 \\ Z^{-1}M_{21}(I - N_{11}^{-1}) & I \end{pmatrix}, \qquad (2.20)
$$

and of course $\beta^* = N^{-1}M\beta$. Noting that $Z = R - (1 + \tau^2)^{-1}rr'$ and substituting the specific forms (2.18) and (2.19) into (2.20) yields the desired result.$\square$

It is easy to check that if $d = 1$, that is only a single precise predictor is considered, then Result 2.6 specializes to Result 2.1. The other specialization of note is the equi-correlated case described in Section 2.2. Here we have $r = (\rho, \dots, \rho)'$ and $R = (1 - \rho)I + \rho J$, where J is the $d \times d$ matrix with every entry being one. Some manipulation reduces (2.17) to

$$
\frac{\beta_1^*}{\beta_1} \;=\; \left(\frac{1}{1 + \tau^2}\right)\left[1 - \frac{\rho^2 \tau^2}{1 + \tau^2}\left\{\frac{d}{1 - \rho} - \frac{d^2 c_{\rho,\tau}}{(1 - \rho)(1 - \rho + d c_{\rho,\tau})}\right\}\right],
$$
$$
(2.21)
$$

where $c_{\rho,\tau} = \rho - \{\rho^2/(1 + \tau^2)\}$. Evaluation of (2.21) yields the multiplicative bias curves in Figure 2.3. Of course when $d = 1$ the unwieldy expression (2.21) reduces to (2.3) from Result 2.1, as must be the case.

2.9.2 Proof of Result 2.2 from Section 2.3

Note that fitted regression coefficients for $\exp(kX)$ or $\exp(kX^*)$ are not changed by linear rescaling of Z, and let $\tilde{Z} = \{Z - E(Z)\}/SD(Z)$. Let β and β^* be the large-sample limiting coefficients from linear regression of Y on $T = (1, e^{kX}, \tilde{Z})'$ and Y on $T^* = (1, e^{kX^*}, \tilde{Z})'$ respectively. Then mimicking the proof of Result 2.6, $M\beta = E(TY)$ and $N\beta^* = E(T^*Y)$, where $M = E(TT')$ and $N = E(T^*T^{*\prime})$. In the former case,

$$
\begin{pmatrix} 1 & E\left(e^{kX}\right) & 0 \\ E\left(e^{kX}\right) & E\left(e^{2kX}\right) & E\left(\tilde{Z}e^{kX}\right) \\ 0 & E\left(\tilde{Z}e^{kX}\right) & 1 \end{pmatrix}\beta \;=\; \begin{pmatrix} E(Y) \\ E\left(Ye^{kX}\right) \\ E\left(Y\tilde{Z}\right) \end{pmatrix}.
$$
$$
(2.22)
$$

Now the normality of $X^*|X$ and the assumption of nondifferential error yields

$$
E\left(e^{kX^*}\right) = \gamma E\left(e^{kX}\right),\; E\left(e^{2kX^*}\right) = \gamma^4 E\left(e^{2kX}\right),\; E\left(\tilde{Z}e^{kX^*}\right) = \gamma E\left(\tilde{Z}e^{kX}\right),
$$

and $E\left(Ye^{kX^*}\right) = \gamma E\left(Ye^{kX}\right)$, where $\gamma = \exp(k^2\sigma^2\tau^2/2)$. Thus β^* satisfies

$$
\begin{pmatrix}
1 & \gamma E\left(e^{kX}\right) & 0 \\
\gamma E\left(e^{kX}\right) & \gamma^4 E\left(e^{2kX}\right) & \gamma E\left(\tilde{Z}e^{kX}\right) \\
0 & \gamma E\left(\tilde{Z}e^{kX}\right) & 1
\end{pmatrix}
\beta^* =
\begin{pmatrix}
E(Y) \\
\gamma E\left(Ye^{kX}\right) \\
E\left(Y\tilde{Z}\right)
\end{pmatrix},
$$

or equivalently

$$
\begin{pmatrix}
1 & \gamma E\left(e^{kX}\right) & 0 \\
E\left(e^{kX}\right) & \gamma^3 E\left(e^{2kX}\right) & E\left(\tilde{Z}e^{kX}\right) \\
0 & \gamma E\left(\tilde{Z}e^{kX}\right) & 1
\end{pmatrix}
\beta^* =
\begin{pmatrix}
E(Y) \\
E\left(Ye^{kX}\right) \\
E\left(Y\tilde{Z}\right)
\end{pmatrix}.
$$

$$(2.23)$$

Thus the left-hand sides of (2.22) and (2.23) are equal, giving an explicit relationship between β^* and β. Solving for β_1^* in terms of β using Cramer's rule gives

$$
\frac{\beta_1^*}{\beta_1} = \frac{Var\left(e^{kX}\right) - E\left(\tilde{Z}e^{kX}\right)^2}{\gamma\left\{Var\left(e^{kX}\right) - E\left(\tilde{Z}e^{kX}\right)^2\right\} + (\gamma^3 - \gamma)E\left(e^{2kX}\right)}.
$$

Upon noting that

$$
Var\left(e^{kX}\right) - E\left(e^{kX}\tilde{Z}\right)^2 = Var\left(e^{kX}\right)\left[1 - Cor\left(e^{kX}, Z\right)^2\right],
$$

the desired result follows immediately.□

2.9.3   A Result on the Impact of Measurement Error in Logistic Regression Estimates

The following result supports the developments in Section 2.6.

Result 2.7 *Let Y be a 0-1 random variable and let T and T^* be random vectors each with d components and finite means. Let β be the large-sample limiting coefficients from logistic regression of Y on T, and let β^* be the large-sample limiting coefficients from logistic regression of Y on T^*. If $E(T^*|T,Y) = MT$ for some fixed $d \times d$ matrix M, then β^* and β satisfy*

$$
E\left[T^*\left\{\frac{1}{1+\exp(-\beta'T)} - \frac{1}{1+\exp(-\beta^{*'}T^*)}\right\}\right] = 0. \qquad (2.24)
$$

Proof of Result 2.7. Let $g(z) = \{1 + \exp(-z)\}^{-1}$. Under the stated conditions,

$$
\begin{aligned}
E\left[T^*\left\{g(\beta'T) - g(\beta^{*'}T^*)\right\}\right] &= E\left[T^*\left\{Y - g(\beta'T)\right\}\right] \\
&= E\left[E(T^*|T,Y)\left\{Y - g(\beta'T)\right\}\right] \\
&= M\,E\left[T\left\{Y - g(\beta'T)\right\}\right] \\
&= 0,
\end{aligned}
$$

where the first equality follows from (2.13) and the last equality follows from (2.12).□

It is straightforward to verify that the conditions in Result 2.7 are met in all three examples discussed in Section 2.6. The form of (2.24) then suggests an easy approach to approximating β^* for a given β. In particular, let $(T_{(1)}, T_{(1)}^*), \ldots, (T_{(m)}, T_{(m)}^*)$ denote a Monte Carlo sample of m independent draws from the joint distribution of (T, T^*), with m taken to be very large. For a given β, define $\tilde{Y}_{(i)} = \{1 + \exp(-\beta' T_{(i)})\}^{-1}$. Then the value of β^* solving (2.24) can be approximated by the solution to

$$\sum_{i=1}^{m} T_{(i)}^* \left\{ \tilde{Y}_{(i)} - \frac{1}{1 + \exp(-\beta^{*\prime} T_{(i)}^*)} \right\} = 0. \qquad (2.25)$$

This is precisely the form of the logistic regression maximum likelihood equations when $\tilde{Y}_{(i)}$ and $T_{(i)}^*$ are respectively the response variable and the explanatory variables for the i-th case. Of course $\tilde{Y}_{(i)}$ is not binary as per a 'real' logistic regression response variable, but many standard software routines for logistic regression will solve these equations regardless of whether the inputted values of the response variable are binary or not. Thus the value of β^* solving (2.25) is easily obtained from standard software.

CHAPTER 3

The Impact of Mismeasured Categorical Variables

Of course many explanatory variables encountered in statistical practice are categorical rather than continuous in nature. Mismeasurement arises for such a variable when the actual and recorded categories for subjects can differ. Fundamentally this *misclassification* differs from measurement error as discussed in Chapter 2, as now the surrogate variable cannot be expressed as a sum of the true variable plus a noise variable. Rather, one must characterize the mismeasurement in terms of *classification probabilities*, i.e., given the true classification, how likely is a correct classification. This chapter focusses primarily on the impact of misclassification in *binary* explanatory variables, with some discussion of *polychotomous* explanatory variables at the end of the chapter. Schemes to ameliorate the impact of misclassification are not considered until Chapter 5. Thus, as with Chapter 2, this chapter's role is to instill qualitative understanding of when unchecked mismeasurement can produce very misleading results. While the respective literatures on misclassification of categorical explanatory variables and measurement error of continuous explanatory variables have few points of contact, this chapter demonstrates considerable similarities between the respective impacts of both these kinds of mismeasurement.

3.1 The Linear Model Case

Consider the relationship between a continuous response variable Y and a binary explanatory variable V, with the latter taken to have a zero/one coding. Since V is binary, without loss of generality we can write

$$E(Y|V) = \alpha_0 + \alpha_1 V. \qquad (3.1)$$

Now say that for study subjects we observe (Y, V^*) rather than (Y, V), where the zero/one variable V^* is an imperfect surrogate for V. Under the assumption of nondifferential misclassification, whereby V^* and Y are conditionally independent given V, the magnitude of the misclassification can be described by the *sensitivity* and *specificity* of V^* as a surrogate for V. With a view to epidemiological applications, we tend to refer to $V = 0$ as 'negative' or 'unexposed,' and $V = 1$ as 'positive' or 'exposed.' Then the sensitivity $SN = Pr(V^* = 1|V = 1)$ is the probability that a true positive is correctly classified, while the specificity $SP = Pr(V^* = 0|V = 0)$ is the probability that a true negative is correctly classified. Thus the extent to which SN and SP are less than one reflects the severity of the misclassification.

Starting from (3.1) and using the nondifferential property yields

$$
\begin{aligned}
E(Y|V^*) &= E\{E(Y|V)|V^*\} \\
&= \alpha_0 + \alpha_1 E(V|V^*) \\
&= \alpha_0 + \alpha_1 V^* Pr(V = 1|V^* = 1) + \\
&\quad \alpha_1(1 - V^*)Pr(V = 1|V^* = 0) \\
&= \alpha_0^* + \alpha_1^* V^*,
\end{aligned}
$$

where

$$
\alpha_0^* = \alpha_0 + \alpha_1 Pr(V = 1|V^* = 0)
$$

and

$$
\frac{\alpha_1^*}{\alpha_1} = 1 - Pr(V = 0|V^* = 1) - Pr(V = 1|V^* = 0). \qquad (3.2)
$$

In terms of estimating α_1 without any correction for misclassification, (3.2) shows that more attenuation results from larger probabilities of misclassification given the apparent classification.

Of course it might seem more natural to express the attenuation the other way around, in terms of sensitivity and specificity which are probabilities of misclassification given the true classification. Towards this, let $r = Pr(V = 1)$ and $r^* = Pr(V^* = 1)$, which can be thought of as the actual and apparent prevalences of exposure in the population at hand. Clearly r^* is a function of (r, SN, SP) given by

$$
\begin{aligned}
r^* &= Pr(V = 1)Pr(V^* = 1|V = 1) + Pr(V = 0)Pr(V^* = 1|V = 0) \\
&= rSN + (1 - r)(1 - SP) \\
&= (1 - SP) + (SN + SP - 1)r.
\end{aligned}
$$

Also, from Bayes theorem we have

$$
\begin{aligned}
Pr(V = 0|V^* = 1) &= \{Pr(V = 0)Pr(V^* = 1|V = 0)\}/Pr(V^* = 1) \\
&= (1 - r)(1 - SP)/r^*,
\end{aligned}
$$

and similarly

$$
Pr(V = 1|V^* = 0) = r(1 - SN)/(1 - r^*).
$$

Substituting into (3.2) gives the attenuation factor as

$$
\begin{aligned}
\frac{\alpha_1^*}{\alpha_1} &= 1 - \frac{(1 - r)(1 - SP)}{r^*} - \frac{r(1 - SN)}{1 - r^*} \\
&= (SN + SP - 1)\frac{r(1 - r)}{r^*(1 - r^*)}, \qquad (3.3)
\end{aligned}
$$

where the second, perhaps more interpretable, equality follows from the first after some algebraic manipulation. In interpreting (3.3) it must be remembered that r^* is a function of (r, SN, SP).

Clearly (3.3) becomes one when $SN = 1$ and $SP = 1$, as must be the case. By taking partial derivatives it is simple to check that (3.3) is increasing in SN for fixed SP and increasing in SP for fixed SN. Thus the effect of misclassification is an attenuating bias, and the attenuation worsens with the severity of the misclassification. To get a sense for the magnitude of the bias, Figure 3.1 gives contour plots of (3.3) as SN and SP vary, for two different values of r. When $r = 0.5$ (left panel), the bias is symmetric in SN and SP, as can be seen by direct inspection of (3.3). The plotted contours reveal that substantial attenuation can occur without the misclassification being very severe. For instance, $SN = SP = 0.9$, which can be interpreted as 10% misclassification, gives $\alpha_1^*/\alpha_1 = 0.8$, interpreted as 20% attenuation. This can be compared to the analogous finding for continuous measurement error in Section 2.1 where 10% measurement error produces only 1% attenuation. Having 10% of all the measurements 'entirely corrupted' in the binary case is clearly much more damaging than having *all* the measurements corrupted by about 10% in the continuous case! We also note from the contour shapes that 'unbalanced' misclassification where SN and SP differ is slightly less damaging than the balanced case of $SN = SP$. For instance, $(SN = 1, SP = 0.8)$ gives $\alpha_1^*/\alpha_1 = 0.833$, corresponding to slightly less attenuation than the $SN = SP = 0.9$ case.

The right panel of Figure 3.1 corresponds to $r = 0.1$, which can be regarded as a 'rare exposure' scenario typifying many epidemiological investigations. Clearly the attenuation worsens much more with declining specificity than with declining sensitivity in this scenario. This makes sense, as there are far more true negatives than true positives in the population. Hence the specificity describing the classification of true negatives has a bigger impact than the sensitivity describing the classification of true positives. When SN and SP are comparable, the attenuation is now stronger than in the $r = 0.5$ case of common exposure. For instance, $SN = SP = 0.9$ now yields a very strong attenuation factor of 0.49, compared to 0.8 in the $r = 0.5$ case. This is of particular concern in light of the general epidemiological interest in rare exposures. Indeed, still considering $SN = SP = 0.9$ we find from (3.3) that when $r = 0.05$ the attenuation factor drops further to 0.32, an exceedingly substantial attenuation. In the context of a rare exposure, even mild nondifferential misclassification can lead to wildly misleading inferences if left unchecked.

3.2 More General Impact

From Chapter 2 we know that the bias induced in the regression coefficient for an explanatory variable subject to continuous measurement error is worsened by the presence of an additional precisely measured explanatory variable, provided the two explanatory variables are correlated. The following result gives a comparable finding for misclassification. In line with Chapter 2 we frame the result in terms of comparing large-sample limiting coefficients for the mismeasured and properly measured cases, without regard to how well

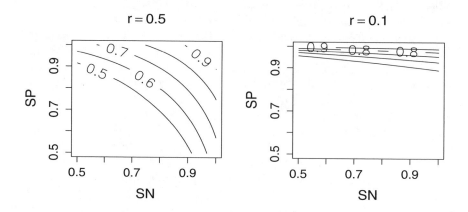

Figure 3.1 *Contours of the attenuation factor as a function of sensitivity and speci-ficity. The left panel corresponds to $r = Pr(V = 1) = 0.5$ and the right panel corresponds to $r = 0.1$. The contours correspond to an attenuation factor (3.3) of 0.9, 0.8, 0.7, 0.6, and 0.5.*

the postulated distribution of the response variable given the explanatory variables matches the actual distribution.

Result 3.1 *Suppose that (Y, V, Z) jointly have finite second moments, where V is a 0-1 random variable. Furthermore, say that V^* is another 0-1 random variable defined according to*

$$Pr(V^* = 1|V, Z, Y) \;=\; a + bV,$$

where

$$a \;=\; 1 - SP,$$
$$b \;=\; SN + SP - 1.$$

That is, we have nondifferential misclassification with sensitivity SN and specificity SP. Let $\alpha = (\alpha_0, \alpha_1, \alpha_2)'$ and $\alpha^* = (\alpha_0^*, \alpha_1^*, \alpha_2^*)'$ be the large-sample limiting coefficients from least-squares regression of Y on $(1, V, Z)'$ and Y on $(1, V^*, Z)'$ respectively. Then,

$$\frac{\alpha_1^*}{\alpha_1} \;=\; b\left[\frac{r(1-r)(1-\rho^2)}{r^*(1-r^*) - r(1-r)\rho^2 b^2}\right], \tag{3.4}$$

$$\alpha_2^* - \alpha_2 \;=\; \alpha_1 \rho \frac{\{r(1-r)\}^{1/2}}{\sigma_z}\left[1 - b\left(\frac{\alpha_1^*}{\alpha_1}\right)\right],$$

$$\alpha_0^* - \alpha_0 \;=\; r\alpha_1 - r^*\alpha_1^* + \mu_z(\alpha_2^* - \alpha_2),$$

where $r = Pr(V = 1)$, $r^* = Pr(V^* = 1) = a + br$, $\mu_z = E(Z)$, $\sigma_z = SD(Z)$, and $\rho = Cor(V, Z)$.

We focus on (3.4), the attenuation factor in estimating the slope α_1 without correction for misclassification. It is straightforward to verify that this factor is increasing in SN for fixed (SP, r, ρ), and increasing in SP for fixed (SN, r, ρ), as is to be expected. In Section 3.8 we also verify that (3.4) is decreasing in $|\rho|$ for fixed SN, SP, and r. That is, the attenuation does worsen with increasing correlation between the two explanatory variables. Note as well that when $\rho = 0$, (3.4) reduces to (3.3). Finally, in Section 3.8 we show that as a function of r for fixed SN, SP, and ρ, the attenuation factor (3.4) is largest when

$$
r = \begin{cases} \frac{SP(1-SP)-\{SP(1-SP)-SN(1-SN)\}^{1/2}}{SP(1-SP)-SN(1-SN)} & \text{if } SN \neq SP, \\ 1/2 & \text{if } SN = SP, \end{cases}
$$

with (3.4) decreasing to zero as r decreases from this value to zero or increases from this value to one. Particularly, the former case again raises concern about an acute impact of misclassification in rare-exposure scenarios.

To convey a more concrete sense of the magnitude of the attenuation, Figure 3.2 gives contour plots of the attenuation factor (3.4) as a function of SN and SP, for selected values of r and ρ. The top two panels in which $\rho = 0$ are identical to Figure 3.1. The lower panels then document the further attenuation that results when the second predictor Z is correlated with V. In particular, the $\rho = 0.5$ scenarios yield slightly more bias than the $\rho = 0$ scenarios, while the $\rho = 0.8$ scenarios evidence considerably more bias. Thus the warning in the previous section about mild misclassification having the potential to induce substantial bias is now even more dire: both rare exposure and correlation between the exposure and additional precisely measured covariate are catalysts for this situation.

3.3 Inferences on Odds-Ratios

We now turn attention to situations where the response variable is also binary. In particular, say both the response Y and predictor V are binary, with no other explanatory variables at play. Adopting a common epidemiological scenario, say that $Y = 1$ indicates the presence of a particular disease, while $V = 1$ indicates exposure to a putative risk. Let

$$
\begin{aligned}
r_0 &= Pr\{V = 1 | Y = 0\}, \\
r_1 &= Pr\{V = 1 | Y = 1\},
\end{aligned}
$$

be the prevalences of exposure amongst disease-free and diseased subjects respectively. As is intuitive and well known, (r_0, r_1) can be estimated from either prospective or retrospective (case-control) studies. Typically, inferential interest would focus on

$$
\Psi = \frac{r_1/(1 - r_1)}{r_0/(1 - r_0)},
$$

the odds-ratio describing the association between exposure and disease.

Now say that V is subject to nondifferential misclassification as in the previous section, with the surrogate exposure variable again denoted by V^*.

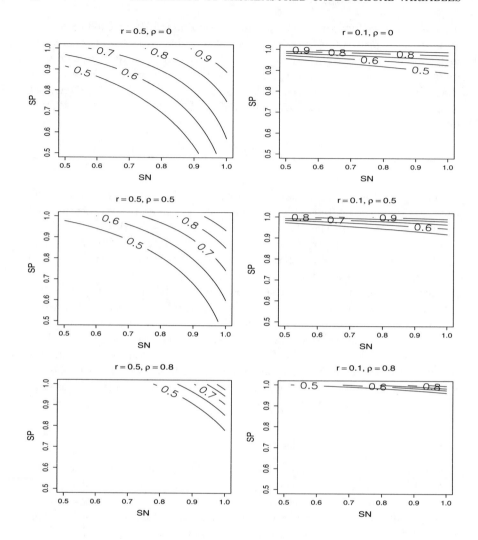

Figure 3.2 *Contours of the attenuation factor as a function of sensitivity and speci-ficity, in the presence of an additional precisely measured explanatory variable. The two columns correspond to $r = 0.5$ and $r = 0.1$, while the three rows correspond to $\rho = 0$, $\rho = 0.5$, and $\rho = 0.8$ The contours correspond to an attenuation factor (3.4) of 0.9, 0.8, 0.7, 0.6, and 0.5.*

Without any adjustment for misclassification, the analyst would infer the exposure prevalences to be $(\tilde{r}_0, \tilde{r}_1)$ in the large-sample limit, where

$$
\begin{aligned}
\tilde{r}_i &= Pr(V^* = 1|Y = i) \\
&= E\{Pr(V^* = 1|V, Y = i)|Y = i\} \\
&= E\{Pr(V^* = 1|V)|Y = i)\} \\
&= Pr(V^* = 1|V = 1)Pr(V = 1|Y = i) + \\
&\quad Pr(V^* = 1|V = 0)Pr(V = 0|Y = i) \\
&= a + br_i,
\end{aligned}
$$

where, as before, $a = 1 - SP$ and $b = SN + SP - 1$. Consequently the large-sample limit of the estimated odds ratio would be

$$
\tilde{\Psi} = \frac{\tilde{r}_1/(1 - \tilde{r}_1)}{\tilde{r}_0/(1 - \tilde{r}_0)}.
$$

After some algebraic manipulations, the attenuation factor that arises from treating V^* as if it were V is

$$
\frac{\tilde{\Psi}}{\Psi} = \frac{\{1 + d/r_1\}/\{1 + c/(1 - r_1)\}}{\{1 + d/r_0\}/\{1 + c/(1 - r_0)\}}, \tag{3.5}
$$

with

$$
c = \frac{1 - SN}{SN + SP - 1}
$$

and

$$
d = \frac{1 - SP}{SN + SP - 1}.
$$

If $SN + SP > 1$, which is a weak condition that might be interpreted as the exposure assessment being more accurate than a coin-flip guess, then it is clear that (3.5) really does correspond to attenuation towards an odds-ratio of unity. That is, either $1 \leq \tilde{\Psi} \leq \Psi$, or $\Psi \leq \tilde{\Psi} \leq 1$.

Though not typically expressed in this fashion, the attenuation factor (3.5), or slight variants thereof, have been derived and discussed by numerous authors; see, for instance, Bross (1954), Goldberg (1975), Barron (1977), and Copeland, Checkoway, McMichael and Holbrook (1977). These articles tend to focus on sample odds-ratios associated with two-by-two exposure-disease tables describing finite samples, rather than large-sample limits. In particular, the odds-ratio for the nominally observed table describing measured exposure and outcome is compared to the nominally unobserved table describing actual exposure and outcome. However, the difference between the finite sample and large-sample views in this context is stylistic at most.

To get a sense for the magnitude of the bias induced by misclassification, Figure 3.3 gives contour plots of the odds-ratio Ψ and the attenuation factor $\tilde{\Psi}/\Psi$, as functions of the prevalences (r_0, r_1). In particular, three such plots for three values of (SN, SP) are given for the attenuation factor. By comparing the plot for the odds-ratio to any of the plots for the attenuation factor, we

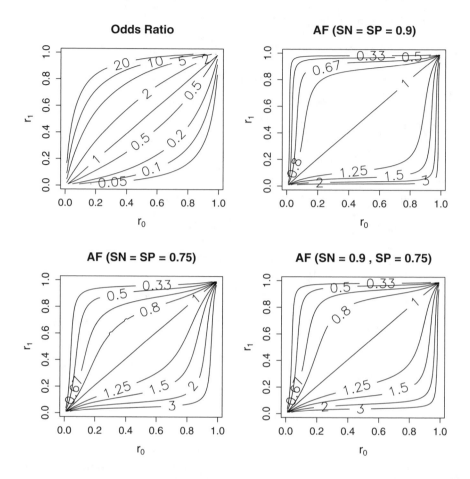

Figure 3.3 *Contours of the odds ratio and attenuation factor as a function of exposure prevalences. The upper-left panel gives contours of the odds-ratio Ψ as a function of exposure prevalences (r_0, r_1). The other three panels give contours of the attenuation factor (3.5) for three combinations of sensitivity and specificity. The upper-right panel corresponds to $(SN, SP) = (0.9, 0.9)$, the lower-left panel corresponds to $(SN, SP) = (0.75, 0.75)$, and the lower right panel corresponds to $(SN, SP) = (0.9, 0.75)$.*

see the attenuation is much more pronounced when the true odds-ratio is far from one. In fact, if we consider a scenario where Ψ tends to infinity (because either r_0 tends to zero for fixed r_1 or r_1 tends to one for fixed r_0), we see that the attenuation factor tends to zero, with $\tilde{\Psi}$ tending to a constant.

Focussing on the mild misclassification scenario involving $SN = SP = 0.9$ in Figure 3.3, we see an attenuation factor of 0.8 when $\Psi > 1$ (or equivalently 1.25 when $\Psi < 1$) can arise without either prevalence or the odds ratio being

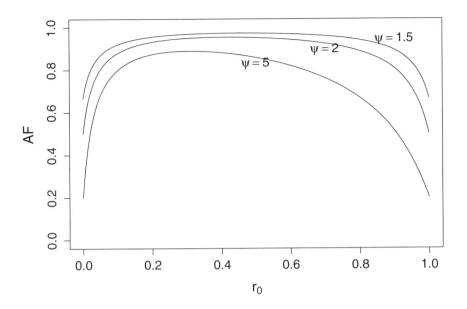

Figure 3.4 *Attenuation factor (3.5) as a function of the prevalence r_0, for some fixed values of the true odds-ratio Ψ. The misclassification is based on $SN = SP = 0.9$. Values $\Psi = 1.5$, $\Psi = 2$, and $\Psi = 5$ are considered.*

particularly extreme. Thus fairly mild misclassification can yield a sizeable inferential bias under plausible conditions. And of course even more substantial bias can arise in the other two scenarios involving larger misclassification probabilities.

To elaborate further, in the $SN = SP = 0.9$ scenario Figure 3.4 displays the attenuation factor (3.5) as a function of r_0, for some fixed values of the true underlying odds ratio Ψ. It is easy to verify from (3.5) that for fixed values of Ψ, SN, and SP, the attenuation factor tends to $1/\Psi$ as r_0 tends to zero or one. That is, perfect attenuation occurs in this limit, with $\tilde{\Psi}$ tending to 1 regardless of the value of Ψ or the extent of the misclassification as reflected by (SN, SP). Moreover, the figure suggests this limit is approached quite rapidly as r_0 goes to zero. Hence inference about the odds ratio can be exquisitely sensitive to even relatively modest misclassification in a rare exposure scenario. There is less attenuation for mid-range prevalences, although the effect is still sizeable. For instance, when $\Psi = 5$ the *largest* value of the attenuation factor is about 0.85 as r_0 varies.

3.4 Logistic Regression

Of course the relatively simple form of (3.5) describes attenuation when the analysis incorporates only the binary outcome variable and the misclassified binary exposure variable. In practice most investigations involve other explanatory variables as well. Thus we turn our attention to scenarios where an additional precisely-measured explanatory variable Z is recorded. For simplicity we consider the scenario where Z is also binary, though the treatment when Z is continuous would be virtually the same.

One approach to investigating the impact of misclassification in this scenario is to consider separate two-by-two (Y, V) tables for the two levels of Z, and then determine the resulting 'typical' (Y, V^*) tables stratified by Z. In particular, odds-ratios in the latter tables can be compared to those in the former. This approach is pursued by Greenland (1980), under various assumptions about the misclassification mechanism. Our related approach is to compare logistic regression of Y on (V^*, Z) to logistic regression of Y on (V, Z), in line with the investigation in Section 2.6 for a continuous exposure variable.

Again we consider nondifferential misclassification, expressed as $Pr(V^* = 1|V, Z, Y) = a + bV$, where $a = 1 - SP$ and $b = SN + SP - 1$. Also, say that the logistic regression model

$$\text{logit}\, Pr(Y = 1|V, Z) \quad = \quad \alpha_0 + \alpha_1 V + \alpha_2 Z \tag{3.6}$$

is postulated for $Y|V, Z$. In particular, this involves the nontrivial assumption that an interaction effect is not manifested.

Whether or not (3.6) is correct, let $\alpha = (\alpha_0, \alpha_1, \alpha_2)'$ be the large-sample limiting coefficients resulting from logistic regression of Y on $T = (1, V, Z)'$. Correspondingly, let α^* be the large-sample limiting coefficients resulting from logistic regression of Y on $T^* = (1, V^*, Z)'$. Adopting the approach detailed in Chapter 2, it is clear that the relationship between α^* and α is governed by the system of three equations

$$g(\alpha) \quad = \quad g^*(\alpha^*), \tag{3.7}$$

where

$$g(\alpha) \quad = \quad E\left\{ \begin{pmatrix} 1 \\ a + bV \\ Z \end{pmatrix} \frac{1}{1 + \exp(-\alpha'T)} \right\},$$

and

$$g^*(\alpha^*) \quad = \quad E\left\{ \begin{pmatrix} 1 \\ V^* \\ Z \end{pmatrix} \frac{1}{1 + \exp(-\alpha^{*\prime}T^*)} \right\}.$$

Note, in particular, that the relationship between α and α^* is the same regardless of the actual response distribution of $Y|V, Z$. Of course similar observations were made in Chapter 2 concerning continuous measurement error.

Given (SN, SP) and the joint distribution of (V, Z), it is straightforward to

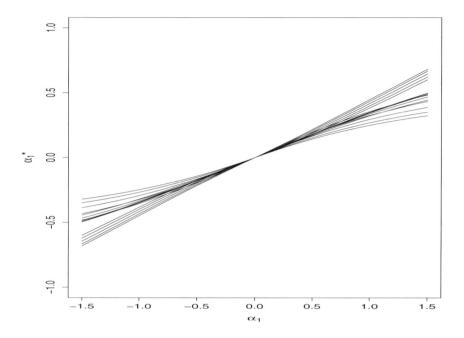

Figure 3.5 *The large-sample coefficient α_1^* for V^* as a function of the large-sample coefficient α_1 for V. The scenario involves $Pr(V = 1) = Pr(Z = 1) = 0.25$, $Cor(V, Z) = 0.5$, $SN = 0.9$, $SP = 0.7$. Each curve is α_1^* plotted against α_1, for fixed values of α_0 and α_2. These values are combinations of $\alpha_0 = -2, 0, 2$ and $\alpha_1 = -1, -0.5, 0, 0.5, 1$.*

evaluate $g(\alpha)$. Moreover, the joint distribution of (V^*, Z) is easily determined, so that g^* and its first derivative can be computed. Consequently, for a given α one can find the value of α^* solving (3.7) via the Newton-Raphson method.

Of course for linear models with either continuous nondifferential measurement error or binary nondifferential misclassification we have seen the effect on the coefficient of interest to be the same multiplicative attenuation regardless of the underlying values of the coefficients. For instance, the attenuation factor (α_1^*/α_1) given in (3.4) does not depend on α. Based on numerical investigation we find this to be *approximately* true in the present situation. To illustrate, consider a scenario under which $Pr(V = 1) = Pr(Z = 1) = 0.25$, $Cor(V, Z) = 0.5$, $SN = 0.9$, $SP = 0.7$. For a variety of values of α_0 and α_2 we plot α_1^* as a function of α_1 in Figure 3.5. We see that the relationship passes through the origin and is quite close to linear, with some modest curvature for large values of α_1. We also see that the slope of the near-linear relationship varies only slightly with α_0 and α_2. Thus the attenuation factor only varies slightly with $\alpha = (\alpha_0, \alpha_1, \alpha_2)'$.

In light of the insensitivity of the attenuation factor to the underlying co-

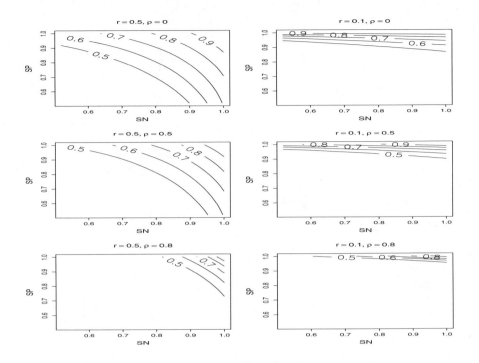

Figure 3.6 *Contours of the attenuation factor* (α_1^*/α_1) *as a function of sensitivity and specificity under logistic regression. The columns correspond to values of* 0.5 *and* 0.1 *for* $q = Pr(V = 1) = Pr(Z = 1)$. *The rows correspond to values of* 0, 0.5, *and* 0.8 *for* $\rho = Cor(V, Z)$. *Within each panel the contours correspond to attenuation factors of* 0.9, 0.8, 0.7, 0.6, *and* 0.5. *The underlying large-sample limiting coefficients are* $\alpha = (-1, 0.5, 0.25)'$.

efficients, we arbitrarily fix $\alpha = (-1, 0.5, 0.25)$ and give contour plots of the attenuation factor (α_1^*/α_1) as a function of SN and SP. This is done for combinations of $Pr(V = 1) = Pr(Z = 1) = 0.5$ or $Pr(V = 1) = Pr(Z = 1) = 0.1$, and $Cor(V, Z) = 0$, $Cor(V, Z) = 0.5$, or $Cor(V, Z) = 0.8$. These plots, which appear in 3.6, bear a striking similarity to those in Figure 3.2. That is, the bias induced by nondifferential misclassification in logistic regression is very similar to that induced in linear regression. A similar finding for nondifferential continuous measurement error was commented upon in Chapter 2.

3.5 Differential Misclassification

Of course the assumption that misclassification is nondifferential is not benign. In case-control analysis particularly there is concern about recall bias inducing misclassification which is actually differential. Say, for instance, that the binary exposure measurement is obtained from a questionnaire administered to subjects, perhaps with the potential exposure occurring years prior to the administration of the questionnaire. Under such circumstances a subject's disease status might have a subtle influence on his recall about the possible past exposure. While it is almost impossible to say anything general about the bias arising in such differential settings, one can give some example scenarios. We do so in the simple setting of having no additional precisely measured explanatory variables. In particular, the apparent exposure prevalences $\tilde{r}_0$ and $\tilde{r}_1$ given by (3.8) are modified to

$$\tilde{r}_i = r_i SN_i + (1 - r_i)(1 - SP_i), \qquad (3.8)$$

so that both the sensitivity and specificity of the exposure assessment may differ for controls ($i = 0$) and cases ($i = 1$). As before, of course, an analysis which ignores misclassification will be estimating the odds-ratio based on $(\tilde{r}_0, \tilde{r}_1)$ rather than the desired odds-ratio based on (r_0, r_1).

To investigate further we consider two scenarios. The first involves true exposure prevalences $(r_0, r_1) = (0.15, 0.22)$, while the second involves $(r_0, r_1) = (0.025, 0.0395)$. In both cases the true odds ratio is $\Psi = 1.6$, but clearly the latter scenario involves a much rarer exposure than the former. Each prevalence scenario in considered in tandem with three misclassification scenarios. The first is simply mild nondifferential misclassification with $SN_0 = SN_1 = 0.9$ and $SP_0 = SP_1 = 0.9$. The second, labelled as the 'denial' scenario, involves cases being slightly more reticent than controls to admit being exposed. Clearly this might arise if the exposure is of a self-inflicted nature, as cases may be wary of interpretations whereby their actions have contributed to their disease. Particularly, we take $SP_0 = SP_1 = 0.9$, but $SN_0 = 0.95$ and $SN_1 = 0.85$ for this scenario. On the other hand, scenarios where cases might be differentially tempted to falsely claim exposure, so as to explain or attribute blame for their plight, are also plausible. In this 'blame' scenario we take $SN_0 = SN_1 = 0.9$, but $SP_0 = 0.95$ and $SP_1 = 0.85$.

Limiting odds-ratios under these scenarios appear in Table 3.1. Clearly differential misclassification can either attenuate or accentuate the actual odds-ratio, with the denial misclassification leading to stronger attenuation than the nondifferential misclassification, but the blame misclassification leading to accentuation of the effect. It is interesting to note that for all three misclassification scenarios there is more bias when exposure is rarer. This is very much in keeping with the other scenarios considered in this chapter.

3.6 Polychotomous Variables

Another situation where the impact of misclassification is complex and hard to intuit is when a polychotomous (i.e., categorical with more than two levels) exposure variable is subject to misclassification. As pointed out by Dosemeci, Wacholder and Lubin (1990), even the impact of nondifferential misclassification can be quite unpredictable in this scenario. Birkett (1992) and Weinberg, Umbach and Greenland (1994) shed further light on this issue. Here we provide a very simple example to illustrate that nondifferential misclassification of a

prevalences	misclassification	apparent OR
(0.15, 0.22)	none	1.60
	nondifferential	1.35
	differential - "denial"	1.23
	differential - "blame"	2.13
(0.025, 0.0395)	none	1.60
	nondifferential	1.11
	differential - "denial"	1.08
	differential - "blame"	2.85

Table 3.1 *Bias in odds-ratio for case-control study with various misclassification scenarios. The nondifferential scenario involves $SN = SP = 0.9$. The "denial" scenario involves $SP = 0.9$, but $SN_0 = 0.95$ for controls and $SN_1 = 0.85$ for cases. The "blame" scenario involves $SN = 0.9$, but $SP_0 = 0.95$ for controls and $SP_1 = 0.85$ for cases.*

polychotomous explanatory variable does not necessarily lead to attenuation in the exposure-disease relationship.

Consider a continuous response variable Y and a polychotomous exposure variable V which takes on one of k values. For simplicity we use $1, \ldots, k$ to label these levels. Now say that nondifferential misclassification gives rise to V^* as a surrogate for V. Let $\gamma_j = E(Y|V = j)$ and $\gamma_j^* = E(Y|V^* = j)$. A straightforward probability calculation then yields

$$\gamma_j^* = \frac{\sum_{i=1}^k \gamma_i Pr(V^* = j|V = i)Pr(V = i)}{\sum_{i=1}^k Pr(V^* = j|V = i)Pr(V = i)}. \quad (3.9)$$

Numerical experimentation with (3.9) quickly indicates that the impact of misclassification is no longer very predictable or intuitively clear. In particular, one can construct plausible scenarios where the impact of nondifferential misclassification is not necessarily attenuation. For instance, say $k = 3$, with the ordered levels $V = 1$, $V = 2$, and $V = 3$ corresponding to no exposure, mild exposure, and substantial exposure respectively. Say that V is uniformly distributed across the three categories, while $V^*|V$ is distributed as

$$Pr(V^* = j|V = i) = \begin{pmatrix} 0.7 & 0.2 & 0.1 \\ 0.15 & 0.7 & 0.15 \\ 0.1 & 0.2 & 0.7 \end{pmatrix},$$

where i indexes rows and j indexes columns of the matrix. Clearly this distribution of $V^*|V$ has plausible characteristics. In particular, when $V = 1$ or $V = 3$ the chance of the classification being off by two categories is less than the chance of being off by just one category. Also, for each value of V the probability of correct classification is relatively large.

Now say that $E(Y|V)$ is given by $\gamma = (0, 0.25, 3)'$. Then calculation via (3.9) gives $\gamma^* = (0.355, 0.705, 2.25)'$. Note, in particular, that $\gamma_2^* - \gamma_1^* = 0.349$

is larger than $\gamma_2 - \gamma_1 = 0.25$. That is, the *apparent* effect of mild exposure relative to no exposure is larger than the actual effect. Clearly attenuation does not always result from nondifferential misclassification of polychotomous explanatory variables. As noted by Carroll (1997), situations where plausible measurement error leads to accentuation of effects are quite unusual and curious!

3.7 Summary

In some broad sense this chapter has conveyed a similar story to that of Chapter 2. Nondifferential misclassification of a binary explanatory variable yields attenuated estimates of associated effects, as does nondifferential measurement error in a continuous explanatory variable. While binary misclassification seems to be more damaging than continuous measurement error in general, they share some key features. In both cases a primary determinant of how bad the bias will be is the strength of correlation between the mismeasured explanatory variable and other precisely measured explanatory variables. Also, the notion of the mismeasurement bias not depending on the actual distribution of the response variable carries over from the previous chapter.

One feature not in play in Chapter 2 is the prevalence of exposure. Generally speaking the bias due to mismeasurement worsens as the proportion of subjects exposed gets close to zero (or close to one). In epidemiological contexts it is often quite natural to conduct studies with low exposure prevalences, so there is a clear need for methods which can adjust inferences to account for misclassification. Such methods are considered in Chapter 5, after methods which adjust for continuous measurement error are discussed in the next chapter.

3.8 Mathematical Details

To show that the attenuation factor (3.4) decreases with $|\rho|$, note that direct differentiation of (3.4) with respect to ρ^2 shows this to be the case provided that

$$b^2 r(1-r) \quad < \quad r^*(1-r^*).$$

Using $r^* = (1 - SP) + (SN + SP - 1)r$, the inequality can be rewritten as

$$(SN + SP - 1)(SN - SP)r \quad < \quad SP(1 - SP). \tag{3.10}$$

We focus on the nonpathological case of better-than-chance assessment, i.e., $SN + SP > 1$, while also assuming that both SN and SP are strictly less than one. Then (3.10) holds trivially if $SN \leq SP$. If $SN > SP$ then the left-hand side of (3.10) as a function of SN and r is largest when $r = 1$ and SN tends to one, with equality obtained in the limit. Thus we have determined that the attenuation factor is decreasing in $|\rho|$, i.e., the attenuation worsens as correlation between the two explanatory variables increases.

Also we wish to establish the behaviour of the attenuation factor (3.4) as a function of prevalence r for fixed SN, SP, and ρ. Upon noting that (3.4) is a ratio of quadratic functions of r, direct differentiation reveals the derivative of (3.4) with respect to r has the same sign as

$$g(r) \quad = \quad (SN + SP - 1)(SN - SP)r^2 - 2SP(1 - SP)r + SP(1 - SP),$$

regardless of the value of ρ. It is straightforward to check that $g()$ is decreasing and must cross zero on $(0, 1)$. If $SN = SP$ then clearly $r = 1/2$ is the solution to $g(r) = 0$. If $SN \neq SP$ then the quadratic formula gives the solution as

$$r \quad = \quad \frac{SP(1 - SP) - \{SP(1 - SP)SN(1 - SN)\}^{1/2}}{SP(1 - SP) - SN(1 - SN)},$$

as desired, where we have used the algebraic fact that $(SN + SP - 1)(SN - SP) = SP(1 - SP) - SN(1 - SN)$ in obtaining this expression.

CHAPTER 4

Adjusting for Mismeasured Continuo Variables

Having discussed at length the deleterious impact of treating mismeasured explanatory variables as if they are precisely measured, we now turn to methods of analysis which recognize and adjust for such mismeasurement. This chapter considers adjustments for the mismeasurement of continuous explanatory variables. Whereas the discussion in Chapters 2 and 3 about the performance of naive estimation in the presence of mismeasurement applies to different methods of statistical inference, we now turn to Bayesian inference implemented with MCMC algorithms as a route to adjust for mismeasurement. Readers with little background in the Bayes-MCMC approach are advised to consult the Appendix, and perhaps some of the references cited therein, before delving into what follows.

4.1 Posterior Distributions

In line with earlier chapters, let Y be the outcome or response variable, let X be the true value of a continuous explanatory variable which is subject to measurement error, let X^* be the noisy measurement of X, and let Z be a vector of other explanatory variables which are precisely measured. If the measurement error mechanism is viewed in terms of the distribution of the surrogate X^* given the true X, it is natural to factor the joint density of the relevant variables as

$$f(x^*, y, x, z) = f(x^*|y, x, z)f(y|x, z)f(x|z)f(z). \qquad (4.1)$$

The first term on the right in (4.1), the conditional density of $(X^*|Y, X, Z)$, can be called the *measurement model*. This describes how the surrogate explanatory variable X^* arises from the true explanatory variable X, with Y and Z possibly influencing this process. The second term for $(Y|X, Z)$, which we refer to as the *outcome model* or the *response model*, describes the relationship between the response variable Y and the actual explanatory variables (X, Z). Typically the primary inferential goal is to uncover the form of this relationship. Taken together, the third and fourth terms give the joint distribution of (X, Z), which might be referred to as the *exposure model* in epidemiological applications. As we shall see, however, the third term usually plays a more pivotal role than the fourth term. The terminology of outcome, measurement, and exposure models, or slight variants of this, is fairly common. For instance, Richardson and Gilks (1993a,b) emphasize the trichotomy of disease, measurement, and exposure models, in some of the first work to detail the application of MCMC techniques to Bayesian analysis in measurement error scenarios. Other 'early' work includes Stephens and Dellaportas (1992), Dellaportas and Stephens (1995), and Mallick and Gelfand (1996).

In a parametric modelling framework, specific distributions might be assumed for the components in (4.1), each involving unknown parameters. Then (4.1) guides the construction of a likelihood function, which could be used to make inferences about the unknown parameters if (X^*, Y, X, Z) were observed for each subject. Of course in reality only (X^*, Y, Z) is observed, so that

$$
\begin{aligned}
f(x^*, y, z) &= \int f(x^*, y, x, z) \, dx \\
&= \left\{ \int f(x^*|y, x, z) f(y|x, z) f(x|z) \, dx \right\} f(z) \qquad (4.2)
\end{aligned}
$$

is required to form the likelihood. In some problems the integral involved is tractable so that the likelihood function is readily evaluated. In other problems, however, the integral will not have a closed-form. A strength of Bayes-MCMC analysis is that (4.2) is not required explicitly. Instead, we can work with (4.1) and let the MCMC algorithm do the required integration implicitly. A non-Bayes route to explicitly working with (4.1) but implicitly working with (4.2) is provided by the EM algorithm (Dempster, Laird and Rubin 1977), which we will comment upon later in this chapter.

As an example, say that the measurement model is both fully known and nondifferential, so that $f(x^*|y, x, z) = f(x^*|x)$ is a known distribution. This might occur if the measurement error mechanism has been investigated thoroughly in previous external studies. We note in passing, however, that the characteristics of mismeasurement processes are not always stable when the measurement scheme is transported from one population to another. For instance it would not be shocking for $Var(X^*|X)$ to differ when the same physical measurement scheme is applied in two populations with dissimilar characteristics. Thus it is not automatic that one could learn the measurement model with data from one population and use this knowledge when adjusting for mismeasurement in a second population. Another situation where one might want to take the measurement model distribution as known is when in fact the mismeasurement process is poorly understood, and one simply wishes to perform *sensitivity analysis* by doing the analysis under a number of different plausible choices for $f(x^*|x)$. Then interest focusses on the extent to which inferences change as the posited distribution changes.

While $f(x^*|x)$ is taken as known, say the response model $f(y|x, z, \theta_R)$ is only known up to a parameter vector θ_R, while the first component of the exposure model $f(x|z, \theta_{E1})$ is known up to a parameter vector θ_{E1}. It will turn out to be superfluous, but also say that the second component of the exposure model $f(z|\theta_{E2})$ is known up to a parameter vector θ_{E2}. Let $\theta = (\theta_R, \theta_{E1}, \theta_{E2})$ comprise all the unknown parameters involved. Bayesian inference requires a prior distribution for these parameters, which we encapsulate with a prior density $f(\theta_R, \theta_{E1}, \theta_{E2})$. Assuming a study with n subjects whose explanatory variables and outcomes can be regarded as independent of one another, the joint distribution of all the relevant quantities is given as

$$f(x^*, y, x, z, \theta) = \left\{ \prod_{i=1}^{n} f(x_i^*|x_i)f(y_i|x_i, z_i, \theta_R)f(x_i|z_i, \theta_{E1})f(z_i|\theta_{E2}) \right\} \times$$
$$f(\theta_R, \theta_{E1}, \theta_{E2}). \tag{4.3}$$

The 'rough-and-ready' form of Bayes theorem states that the density of unobserved quantities U given observed quantities O is *proportional* to the joint density of U and O, where the proportionality is as a function U, for the actually observed O values. Applying this in the present context with $U = (x, \theta_R, \theta_{E1}, \theta_{E2})$ and $O = (x^*, y, z)$ causes us to recast (4.3) slightly as

$$f(x, \theta|x^*, y, z) \propto \left\{ \prod_{i=1}^{n} f(x_i^*|x_i)f(y_i|x_i, z_i, \theta_R)f(x_i|z_i, \theta_{E1})f(z_i|\theta_{E2}) \right\} \times$$
$$f(\theta_R, \theta_{E1}, \theta_{E2}). \tag{4.4}$$

If we want the actual normalized posterior density of the unobserved quantities given the observed quantities, then we must compute the integral of (4.4) over the unobserved quantities, given the fixed values of the observed quantities. As alluded to above, computing this integral explicitly may be problematic, or even nearly impossible. However, (4.4) is enough to implement Bayes-MCMC inference. In particular, so long as we can evaluate the right-side of (4.4), we can implement a MCMC algorithm to draw a Monte Carlo sample from the distribution of the unobserved quantities given the observed quantities. Moreover, such a sample for $(x, \theta|x^*, y, z)$ trivially leads to a sample for $(\theta|x^*, y, z)$ upon ignoring the sampled X values. That is, a Monte Carlo sample from the distribution of the unobserved *parameters* given all the observed data is obtained. All inferences about the parameters, and hence about the distributions they describe, stem from this Monte Carlo sample. This is a general strength of Bayes-MCMC inference in problems involving mismeasured, missing, or censored variables. The ideal but unobserved 'complete' data can be treated as unknowns described by the posterior distribution, in order to get at the posterior distribution of the unknown parameters given the observed data.

It is important to note that if θ_{E2} is independent of (θ_R, θ_{E1}) *a priori*, then the same will be true *a posteriori*, as (4.4) can be factored into a term not containing θ_{E2} and a term not containing the other unknowns $(x, \theta_R, \theta_{E1})$. That is,

$$f(x, \theta_R, \theta_{E1}, \theta_{E2}|x^*, y, z) = f(x, \theta_R, \theta_{E1}|x^*, y, z)f(\theta_{E2}|z),$$

where

$$f(x, \theta_R, \theta_{E1}|x^*, y, z) \propto \left\{ \prod_{i=1}^{n} f(x_i^*|x_i)f(y_i|x_i, z_i, \theta_R)f(x_i|z_i, \theta_{E1}) \right\} \times$$
$$f(\theta_R, \theta_{E1}), \tag{4.5}$$

and

$$f(\theta_{E2}|z) \quad \propto \quad \left\{\prod_{i=1}^{n} f(z_i|\theta_{E2})\right\} f(\theta_{E2}). \tag{4.6}$$

We also note that prior independence of (θ_R, θ_{E1}) and θ_{E2} is commonly assumed, in the absence of any plausible reason why prior views about these different sets of parameters ought to be linked. Indeed, commonly a prior of the form

$$f(\theta_R, \theta_{E1}, \theta_{E2}) \quad = \quad f(\theta_R)f(\theta_{E1})f(\theta_{E2})$$

is postulated. As a practical matter then, unless there is specific interest in the distribution of the precisely measured covariates Z, one can dispense with a model for them. One can simply work with (4.5) and not make any modelling assumptions about Z. There is no need to specify $f(z|\theta_{E2})$ or apply MCMC to (4.6). A *conditional exposure model* for the unobserved X given the observed Z suffices for making inferences about the parameters of the response model.

Before proceeding to a second example of determining a posterior distribution from disease, measurement, and exposure models, we pause to consider issues of parameter identifiability in such settings. If the measurement model also involves unknown parameters θ_M, then $\theta = (\theta_M, \theta_R, \theta_{E1})$ constitutes all the unknown parameters at play. Following the formal statistical definition of identifiability, the problem is said to be *identifiable* provided that different values of θ cannot correspond to the same distribution of *observable* data. Otherwise, the problem is said to be *nonidentifiable*. Usually in identifiable situations, *consistent* parameter estimation can be achieved, in the sense that Bayesian or maximum likelihood estimates will converge to true parameter values as the sample size increases. On the other hand, in nonidentifiable situations it may be that no amount of data can lead to the true parameter values, if in fact the true distribution of observable data corresponds to more than one set of parameter values.

In many measurement error scenarios one might like to start with quite general and flexible measurement, response, and exposure models. Typically this would lead to identifiability if all of (X^*, Y, X, Z) are to be observed, but result in nonidentifiability in the actual scenario where only (X^*, Y, Z) are observed. Roughly speaking, some additional knowledge or additional data are needed to gain identifiability. In the example above the extra information is complete knowledge of the measurement model (i.e., no unknown parameters are involved), and virtually any reasonable specification of response and conditional exposure models will yield consistent estimators of θ_R and θ_{E1} based on (4.5). It is not always so easy to verify this mathematically, however, as the distribution of the observable data may not have a closed-form expression.

Two other examples of how identifiability might be realized are considered below, namely having actual measurements of X and X^* for some subset of the study sample, or having repeated measurements of X^* for some subjects. Intuitively, if one wishes to adjust for mismeasurement then one must have some knowledge about how the mismeasurement arises in the sense of how X^*

is distributed given X and possibly (Y, Z), or have some means of learning about this distribution from data. Consideration of identifiability in modelling mismeasurement seems crucial, as in many practical situations one would like to adjust for mismeasurement without having a great deal of knowledge about the mechanisms leading to this mismeasurement. If one pushes too far in this direction, nonidentifiability will come into play.

An interesting facet of Bayesian inference is that in one sense it 'works' whether or not one has parameter identifiability. That is, the mechanics of forming a posterior distribution and obtaining parameter estimates from this distribution can be carried out equally well in nonidentifiable situations, modulo some technical concerns about MCMC which are alluded to in Chapter 5. Of course in another sense no form of inference can work in a nonidentifiable model, as estimators which tend to true parameter values do not result. One intuitive way of thinking about Bayesian inference in the absence of parameter identifiability is that the prior distribution plays more of a role than usual in determining the posterior belief about the parameters having seen the data. The question of whether Bayesian inferences based on nonidentifiable models might sometimes be useful has received scant attention in the literature (but see Neath and Samaniego 1997, and Gustafson, Le and Saskin 2001). A close look at this issue with reference to mismeasurement modelling appears in Section 6.3. In essence it seems that in some mismeasurement scenarios Bayesian inference from a nonidentifiable model can be worthwhile, as often the extent of nonidentifiability is modest, while the available prior information is sufficiently good.

As a second example of constructing a posterior distribution in a measurement error scenario, say that the nondifferential measurement model is only known up to a parameter vector θ_M, but for a randomly selected subset of the study subjects X itself is measured, in addition to (X^*, Y, Z). Commonly this is referred to as a *validation* study design. The subjects with (X^*, Y, X, Z) measurements are called the *complete* cases or the *validation substudy*, while subjects with only (X^*, Y, Z) measurements comprise the *reduced* cases. Validation designs are fairly widespread, as for some exposures it is possible to make *gold-standard* measurements, but this process is too expensive to be used for anything more than a small minority of study subjects. An obvious interesting question involving a cost-information tradeoff is what proportion of the subjects should be selected for gold-standard measurements. See Greenland (1988) and Spiegelman (1994) for discussion on this question.

As before, let θ_R parameterize the response model describing $(Y|X, Z)$, and let θ_{E1} parameterize the conditional exposure model describing $(X|Z)$. Let subscripts c and r denote complete and reduced cases respectively, so that $x = (x_1, \ldots, x_n)$ can be partitioned into x_c and x_r. The posterior density for the unobserved quantities given the observed quantities then takes the form

$$f\left(x_r, \theta_M, \theta_R, \theta_{E1}|x^*, y, x_c, z\right) \quad \propto \quad \prod_{i=1}^{n} f(x_i^*|x_i, \theta_M) \times$$

$$\prod_{i=1}^{n} f(y_i|x_i, z_i, \theta_R) \times$$

$$\prod_{i=1}^{n} f(x_i|z_i, \theta_{E1}) \times$$

$$f(\theta_M, \theta_R, \theta_{E1}). \tag{4.7}$$

Again this is derived from the rough-and-ready version of Bayes theorem which states that the conditional density of all the unobserved quantities given all the observed quantities is proportional to the joint density of the observed and unobserved quantities, viewed as a function of the unobserved quantities with the observed quantities fixed. While the right-hand side of (4.7) does not appear to distinguish between the observed and unobserved components of x, we shall see that MCMC sampling from (4.7) does provide a principled way to make simultaneous inferences about θ_M, θ_R, and θ_{E1}.

As a third scenario, say that no gold standard observations are available, but repeated measurements of X^* are made for at least some study subjects. In particular, say that m_i replicate measurements are made for the i-th subject. If we retain the nondifferential measurement error model parameterized by θ_M, and make the assumption that the replicate measurements of X^* are conditionally independent given the true value of X, then the posterior density of unobserved quantities given observed quantities takes the form

$$f(x, \theta_M, \theta_R, \theta_{E1}|x^*, y, z) \quad \propto \quad \prod_{i=1}^{n} \prod_{j=1}^{m_i} f(x_{ij}^*|x_i, \theta_M) \times$$

$$\prod_{i=1}^{n} f(y_i|x_i, z_i, \theta_R) \times$$

$$\prod_{i=1}^{n} f(x_i|z_i, \theta_{E1}) \times$$

$$f(\theta_M, \theta_R, \theta_{E1}). \tag{4.8}$$

Here x_{ij}^* is the j-th of the m_i replicated X^* measurements for the i-th subject. It is worth noting that assessment of whether the replicates really are conditionally independent given X is a difficult task, given that X is unobserved. Typically this cannot be verified empirically, and thus devolves to consideration of scientific plausibility in the subject-area context at hand.

4.2 A Simple Scenario

We start with a simple example where the constituent models are based on the normal distribution. In particular, the nondifferential measurement model parameterized by $\theta_M = \tau^2$ is

$$X^*|X, Z, Y \sim N(X, \tau^2),$$

the response model parameterized by $\theta_R = (\beta_0, \beta_1, \beta_2, \sigma^2)$ is

$$Y|X, Z \;\sim\; N(\beta_0 + \beta_1 X + \beta_2 Z, \sigma^2),$$

and the conditional exposure model parameterized by $\theta_{E1} = (\alpha_0, \alpha_1, \lambda^2)$ is

$$X|Z \;\sim\; N(\alpha_0 + \alpha_1 Z, \lambda^2).$$

We consider two possible study designs, each involving $n = 250$ subjects. In the first design (X^*, Y, Z) are observed for all subjects, while in addition a gold-standard measurement of X is made for 10 randomly-selected subjects. In the second design, no gold-standard measurements are available, but two replicate measurements of X^* are made for each subject, with the replicates being conditionally independent given the unobserved X.

To proceed we need a prior distribution for all the unknown parameters $(\alpha, \beta, \lambda^2, \sigma^2, \tau^2)$. Without a compelling reason to do otherwise, we assume prior independence of the parameters, so that

$$f(\alpha, \beta, \lambda^2, \sigma^2, \tau^2) \;=\; f(\alpha)f(\beta)f(\lambda^2)f(\sigma^2)f(\tau^2).$$

For the sake of convenience we assign improper 'locally uniform' priors to the regression coefficients β in the outcome model and α in the exposure model. That is, $f(\alpha) \propto 1$ and $f(\beta) \propto 1$. Intuitively, these represent 'prior ignorance' about the parameters, as they do not favour any particular value of the coefficients.

We note that improper priors are not without controversy, and some would prefer to represent prior ignorance with proper but very diffuse distributions. Indeed, improper priors can be problematic for variance parameters. Considerations of mathematical invariance suggest that if ν^2 is an unknown variance then the appropriate notion of a 'flat' prior is $f(\nu^2) \propto \nu^{-2}$, or equivalently $f(\nu) \propto \nu^{-1}$, rather than $f(\nu) \propto 1$. Roughly speaking, however, for such a prior to lead to a proper posterior distribution, it is necessary for the data to absolutely rule out the possibility that $\nu = 0$. Otherwise, the singularity in the prior at $\nu = 0$ will be transferred to the posterior distribution, making it improper. This is a fatal flaw, as it leaves no sense of posterior probability on which to base inferences. To be more specific, consider the second of the study designs. The observed data will definitely rule out $\tau^2 = 0$, as the replicate X^* measurements for a given subject will not be identical. However, since X is not observed, the data will not definitely rule out either $\sigma^2 = 0$ or $\lambda^2 = 0$. Thus improper priors $f(\sigma^2) \propto \sigma^{-2}$ and $f(\lambda^2) \propto \lambda^{-2}$ must be avoided. As a final remark along these lines, MCMC algorithms will not necessarily detect an improper posterior distribution. That is, one can proceed to implement MCMC sampling with a prior that produces an improper posterior, and perhaps obtain output that reasonably purports to represent the posterior distribution, even though the posterior distribution does not exist! Indeed, some early published papers on applications of MCMC methods made exactly this mistake. For more on this problem, see Hobert and Casella (1996).

In light of the foregoing discussion we use proper prior distributions for τ^2, σ^2, and λ^2. For the sake of simple MCMC it is convenient to assign Inverse

Gamma distributions as priors on the variances of normal distributions. We assign the $IG(0.5, 0.5)$ distribution as the prior for each of λ^2, σ^2, and τ^2. As discussed in the Appendix, this choice of hyperparameters can be viewed as giving a 'unit-information' prior, with a prior guess of one for each variance.

The chosen priors have the property of being *conditionally conjugate*, as discussed in the Appendix. For (4.7) in the case of the first study design and (4.8) in the case of the second study design, the *full conditional* distribution of each individual unobserved quantity given the other unobserved quantities and the observed data is easily identified as a standard distribution. For the sake of illustration, these distributions are identified in Section 4.11. The important point is that the ability to simulate draws from these distributions means that a simple MCMC algorithm—the Gibbs sampler—can be used to generate a sample from the joint posterior distribution of all unknowns, either (4.7) or (4.8).

We simulate a synthetic dataset under each study design, taking (X, Z) to have a bivariate normal distribution with standard normal marginal distributions and a 0.75 correlation coefficient. This implies $\alpha_0 = 0$, $\alpha_1 = 0.75$, and $\lambda^2 = 0.4375$. We set $\tau = 0.5$ in the measurement model, corresponding to substantial measurement error relative to $SD(X) = 1$. From Result 2.1 we note that this substantial measurement error will have a considerable impact; naive estimates of β_1 in these circumstances will be considerably biased, with an attenuation factor of 0.64. The parameters in the outcome model are set as $(\beta_0, \beta_1, \beta_2) = (0, 0.5, 0.25)$, and $\sigma = 1$. The datasets for the two designs are taken to be extensions of the same underlying (X^*, Y, Z) data set, with gold-standard measurements for some randomly chosen subjects added under the first design, and a second X^* realization for every subject added under the second design. Scatterplots of Y versus X and Y versus the first or only replicate of X^* appear in Figure 4.1. The superimposed least-squares fits (of Y to X and Y to X^*, ignoring Z in each case) show that attenuation is manifested, though by ignoring Z we do not see the considerable extent to which attenuation is actually at play.

For each study design a posterior sample of size 10000 is simulated, using the Gibbs sampler with 1000 burn-in iterations. That is, a total of 11000 iterations are used. As discussed in the Appendix, for successful Bayesian inference via MCMC sampling, one needs the sampler to both *converge* (i.e., burn-in) within a reasonable number of iterations and exhibit reasonable *mixing* in the sense of rapidly moving around the parameter space once convergence is attained. To garner some sense of how well the Gibbs sampler is working for the particular models and datasets at hand, Figure 4.2 gives traceplots of the Gibbs sampler output for some of the unknowns. These plots indicate both very quick convergence (well within the alloted 1000 burn-in iterations) and good mixing. Thus any posterior quantities of interest can be computed accurately from the MCMC output. Some general discussion of what are useful posterior quantities for inference and how to obtain them from MCMC output is given in the Appendix.

Figure 4.3 presents the posterior densities of β_0, β_1, β_2, and τ for the data

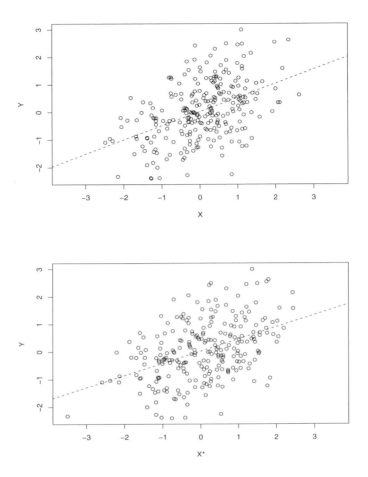

Figure 4.1 *Simulated data in the example of Section 4.2. The top panel is a scatter-plot of Y versus the simulated but nominally unobserved X. The bottom panel is a scatterplot of Y versus the first or only X* replicate. The sample size is n = 250. Each plot includes a least-squares fitted-line, to illustrate the attenuation that results from replacing X with X*.*

sets arising from the two study designs. We also give posterior densities for $(\beta_0, \beta_1, \beta_2)$ under the 'naive' model which assumes the first (or only) X^* replicate is actually a precise measurement of X. Thus we compare inferences which are adjusted for measurement error to those which ignore it. For both study designs we see that the adjustment affects both the location and the width of the posterior densities for β_1 and β_2. As is predictable from the results of Chapter 2, the adjustment shifts the posterior distribution of β_1 away from zero, to correct for attenuation. Also, the effect of adjustment is to

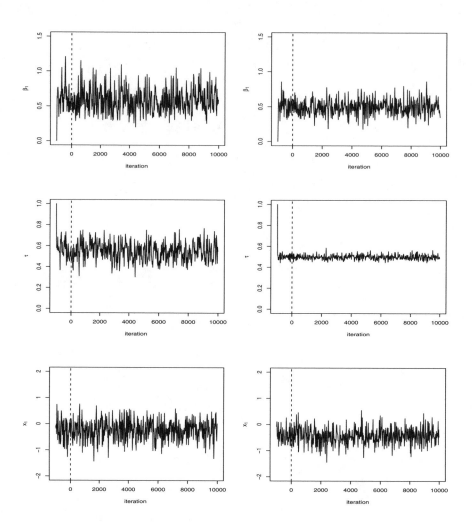

Figure 4.2 *Gibbs sampler output for unknowns β_1, τ, and x_1 in the example of Section 4.2. The plots on the left arise from the first study design, and those on the right from the second study design. The dashed vertical line indicates the end of the allotted burn-in iterations.*

shift the posterior distribution of β_2 toward zero, to compensate for the bias away from zero induced in the coefficient for Z when Z and X are positively correlated. In contrast, the corrected and naive posterior distributions for the intercept β_0 have a common centre. Result 2.1 indicates this is an artifact of X having a distribution which is centred at zero.

Figure 4.3 also shows that after accounting for measurement error the posterior distributions of β_1 and β_2 are wider than their naive counterparts. This

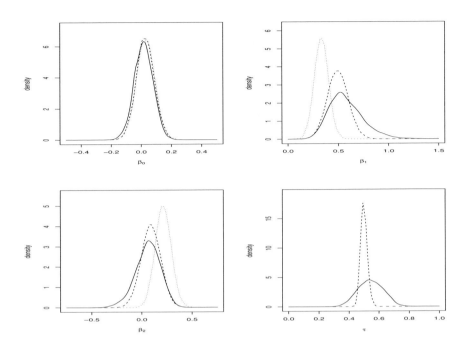

Figure 4.3 *Posterior distributions of β_0, β_1, β_2 and τ in the synthetic data example of Section 4.2. In each case the solid curve gives the posterior density arising from the validation design, the dashed curve gives the posterior density arising from the replication design, and the dotted curve gives the posterior density arising from the naive analysis which treats the first/only replicate of X^* as if it were X.*

extra width correctly reflects the information about X which is lost because only a noisy surrogate X^* is observed. Moreover, we see wider posterior distributions under the validation sample study design than under the replication study design. This arises because the former design, with gold-standard measurements for only 4% of the subjects, contains less information about the measurement model parameter τ than does the replication design. This is directly evidenced by comparing the posterior distribution of τ under the two scenarios. Since the magnitude of the attenuating bias depends on τ, more precise knowledge of τ leads to more precise knowledge of β_1 and β_2. The ability to automatically and appropriately propagate uncertainty from one parameter to another is a strength of the Bayesian approach to inference. An *adhoc* scheme to first determine a point estimate for τ and then use this estimate to derive a bias correction for estimates of β_1 and β_2 would not facilitate such a propagation.

Having carried out Bayes-MCMC analysis for simulated data under these designs, we now point out that in fact this is overkill to some extent. The normal and linear model structures in fact permit explicit determination of the distribution of the outcome Y given the observed explanatory variables X^* and Z, as well as the distribution of X^* given Z. In particular, the jointly normal distribution of (X^*, Y, X) given Z can be identified, and in turn this yields

$$Y|X^*, Z \;\sim\; N\left(\tilde{\beta}_0 + \tilde{\beta}_1 X^* + \tilde{\beta}_2 Z, \tilde{\sigma}^2\right), \tag{4.9}$$

and

$$X^*|Z \;\sim\; N\left(\tilde{\alpha}_0 + \tilde{\alpha}_1 Z, \tilde{\lambda}^2\right), \tag{4.10}$$

where

$$\tilde{\beta}_0 \;=\; \beta_0 + \frac{\alpha_0}{1 + \lambda^2/\tau^2}, \tag{4.11}$$

$$\tilde{\beta}_1 \;=\; \frac{\beta_1}{1 + \tau^2/\lambda^2}, \tag{4.12}$$

$$\tilde{\beta}_2 \;=\; \beta_2 + \frac{\alpha_1 \beta_1}{1 + \lambda^2/\tau^2}, \tag{4.13}$$

$$\tilde{\sigma}^2 \;=\; \sigma^2 + \left(\frac{\lambda^2 \tau^2}{\lambda^2 + \tau^2}\right)\beta_1^2, \tag{4.14}$$

$$\tilde{\alpha}_0 \;=\; \alpha_0, \tag{4.15}$$

$$\tilde{\alpha}_1 \;=\; \alpha_1, \tag{4.16}$$

$$\tilde{\lambda}^2 \;=\; \lambda^2 + \tau^2. \tag{4.17}$$

We call (4.9) and (4.10) the *collapsed model*, as it describes only the observables (X^*, Y, Z) after having marginalized the unobservable X.

Armed with the collapsed model, the likelihood terms for the reduced cases in the validation design can be evaluated directly. Similarly, in the replication design scenario one can easily determine the normal distributions of $Y|X_1^*, X_2^*, Z$ and $X_1^*, X_2^*|Z$. In either design then, the likelihood function for $(\beta_0, \beta_1, \beta_2, \alpha_0, \alpha_1, \tau^2, \sigma^2, \lambda^2)$ can be obtained in closed-form. Hence it is not strictly necessary to use a MCMC algorithm which includes the unobserved values of X as one of the unknown components described by the posterior distribution. The important point, however, is that the MCMC approach is still quite straightforward in problems where a closed-form likelihood function cannot be obtained, as is the situation for the further examples in this chapter.

4.3 Nonlinear Mixed Effects Model: Viral Dynamics

As an example of inferential adjustment for measurement error in the face of a more complex outcome model, we consider a dataset analyzed previously by Wu and Ding (1999), Ko and Davidian (2000) [henceforth KD2000], and Wu (2002) using non-Bayesian techniques. The data describe $n = 44$ HIV-infected patients treated with a combination therapy (ritonavir, 3TC, and zidovudine). Viral load (Plasma HIV-1 RNA) was measured over time for each

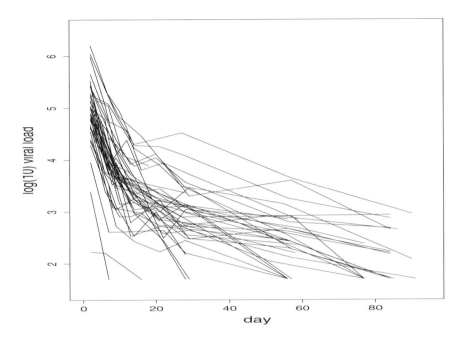

Figure 4.4 *Log_{10} viral load versus day post-treatment for all 44 subjects in the viral load example.*

patient. The number of measurements per patient ranges from two to eight, with the majority of subjects having seven or eight measurements. All but eight subjects had their first measurement on the second day post-treatment, with the exceptions having a first measurement sometime between days three and seven. The duration of follow-up ranges from 7 days to 91 days post-treatment, with a median follow-up of 62 days. To get some sense for the data, Figure 4.4 plots log_{10} viral load versus day post-treatment for all 44 subjects.

The two available covariates which may explain some of the viral dynamics are the baseline viral load and the baseline CD4 cell count. As discussed by KD2000, it is reasonable to view the baseline viral load as a precisely measured explanatory variable, but measured CD4 counts are known to be quite imprecise. There are no gold-standard or replicated measurement of baseline CD4 counts by which to formally gauge the magnitude of the measurement error. Therefore, following KD2000, we simply perform a sensitivity analysis. That is, multiple analyses are performed under different plausible assumptions about the magnitude of the measurement error.

Again following KD2000, the outcome model is

$$\log_{10} Y_{it} \quad \sim \quad N\left(\log_{10} \mu_{it}, \sigma^2\right),$$

where Y_{it} is the viral load for subject i measured on day t. The measurements are considered to be independent across time and across subjects given the underlying means μ_{it}. A typical viral dynamics model gives

$$\mu_{it} = P_{1i}\exp(-\lambda_{1i}t) + P_{2i}\exp(-\lambda_{2i}t),$$

where identifiability is achieved via the constraint $\lambda_{1i} > \lambda_{2i}$. That is, λ_{1i} governs the initial decline in viral load post-treatment, while λ_{2i} affects the longer-term behaviour.

The subject-specific parameters $(P_{1i}, P_{2i}, \lambda_{1i}, \lambda_{2i})$ are expressed in terms of fixed effects $\beta = (\beta_1, \ldots, \beta_7)$ and random effects b_{ki}, $k = 1, \ldots, 4$, $i = 1, \ldots, n$, via

$$\log P_{1i} = \beta_1 + \beta_2 Z_i + b_{1i}, \tag{4.18}$$
$$\log P_{2i} = \beta_3 + \beta_4 Z_i + b_{2i}, \tag{4.19}$$
$$\log \lambda_{1i} = \beta_5 + \beta_6 X_i + b_{3i}, \tag{4.20}$$
$$\log \lambda_{2i} = \beta_7 + b_{4i}. \tag{4.21}$$

Here Z_i and X_i are respectively the baseline $\log_{10}$ viral load and the baseline $\log(CD4/100)$ for the i-th subject. It is self-evident that P_{1i} and P_{2i}, which describe the initial viral load, will be strongly associated with the baseline measurement Z_i via the coefficients β_2 and β_4. The coefficient β_6 describes a hypothesized association between the first-phase decay and the baseline CD4 count.

Still following KD2000, inter-subject variation is modelled by normal distributions for the random effects. That is, all the random effects are considered to be independent of one another, with

$$b_{ki} \sim N(0, \omega_k^2),$$

for $k = 1, \ldots, 4$ and $i = 1, \ldots, n$. In all, the nonlinear mixed effects outcome model is parameterized by $(\beta_1, \ldots, \beta_7, \sigma^2, \omega_1^2, \ldots, \omega_4^2)$. For the purposes of Bayes-MCMC inference, however, we will also include the random effects themselves as unknown quantities described by the posterior distribution.

As mentioned above, the measurement error in Z is thought to be small, and can be ignored. The measurement of X, however, may be subject to substantial error. A nondifferential normal measurement error of the form

$$X^* | Y, X, Z, \sim N(X, \tau^2)$$

is posited. Replicate measurements of X^* are not available, so we simply consider different fixed values of τ in order to conduct a sensitivity analysis. Following KD2000, who in turn were guided by subject-area literature, we use $\tau^2 = 0$, $\tau^2 = 0.12$, $\tau^2 = 0.24$, and $\tau^2 = 0.36$. Since the sample variance of X^* is 0.49, we are entertaining the possibility of very substantial measurement error in X.

Finally, the model specification is completed with an exposure model. Along the lines of the previous example, we take

$$X | Z \sim N(\alpha_0 + \alpha_1 Z, \lambda^2).$$

Of course prior distributions are required for Bayesian analysis. As in the previous example we assign improper locally uniform priors to α and β, but proper priors to the variance components σ^2, ω_1^2, $\ldots$, ω_4^2, and λ^2. Both σ^2 and λ^2 are assigned unit-information inverse gamma prior distributions. Such priors are discussed in the Appendix. In the case of σ^2 the prior guess is $\sigma^2 \approx 4$. This is conservatively large, in the sense that $\sigma = 2$ on the $log_{10} Y_{it}$ scale corresponds to large multiplicative variation on the Y_{it} scale itself. In the case of λ^2 the prior guess is taken to be 0.49, which is the sample variance of X^*. Of course strictly speaking one ought not to use the data in order to choose the prior, though again we are using a conservatively large prior guess, as $Var(X|Z) < Var(X) < Var(X^*)$.

We could also assign inverse gamma priors to the random effect variances $\omega_1^2, \ldots, \omega_4^2$. Indeed, this is by far the most commonly used distribution for the variance of normally distributed random effects in Bayesian hierarchical models, as it leads to a simple Gibbs sampling update for the variance component. Arguably, however, the shape of an inverse gamma density is not appropriate for a random effect variance. In particular, the density goes to zero as the variance goes to zero, so that a variance equal to zero is ruled out *a priori*. However, because the random effects are unobserved, the data do not rule out the possibility that their variance is zero. (In contrast, the data do usually rule out the possibility that the variance of observed quantities given parameters is zero. In linear regression, for instance, if the data are not collinear then the population residual variance cannot be zero.) Indeed, one can show that in a simple random effect model with a random effect variance ω^2 being the only unknown parameter, the likelihood for $\omega^2 = 0$ is positive, and for some datasets the likelihood decreases monotonically as ω^2 increases. In such a case an inverse gamma prior will result in a posterior distribution for ω^2 that has an entirely different shape (increasing from zero to a mode, then decreasing) than the likelihood function. This deficiency of inverse gamma priors for variance components is discussed at more length by Gustafson and Wasserman (1996).

In light of this point, Gustafson (1997, 1998) advocates the use of a half-Cauchy prior for either a random effect variance ω^2 or standard deviation ω. The 'half' simply refers to the truncation of a Cauchy distribution centred at zero to positive values, given that a variance cannot be negative. This form lets the shape of the posterior distribution on ω adapt to the data; that is, the posterior density can either increase then decrease or be monotonically decreasing. In the present context we take

$$f(\omega_i) = \left(\frac{2}{\pi}\right) \frac{1}{\bar{\omega}_i} \frac{1}{1 + (\omega_i/\bar{\omega}_i)^2}, \tag{4.22}$$

where $\bar{\omega}_i$ is a hyperparameter which must be specified. A rough calibration is that $\omega_i = \bar{\omega}_i$ is half as likely as $\omega_i = 0$ according to the prior density (4.22). Based on this, setting each $\bar{\omega}_i = 1$ for $i = 1, \ldots, 4$ seems reasonable for the problem at hand. Given the form of (4.18) through (4.21), $\omega_i = 1$ corresponds to very substantial subject-to-subject variation in the viral dynamics, so the choice of hyperparameters corresponds to quite diffuse prior distributions over *a priori* plausible values of the variance components.

On computational grounds a half-Cauchy prior for the variance of normally distributed random effects initially seems less appealing than an inverse gamma prior. In particular, the full conditional distribution does not correspond to a standard distribution. However, Gustafson (1997, 1998) shows that it 'almost' corresponds to a standard distribution, and gives efficient rejection sampling algorithms which take advantage of this fact. In fact, MCMC updating of a variance component is essentially no more difficult under a half-Cauchy prior than under a inverse gamma prior.

While σ^2, λ^2, ω^2, and α are amenable to Gibbs sampling updates, the remaining unknowns x, b, and β are not. Thus random walk Metropolis-Hastings updates are used for these parameters, though it is extremely tedious to tune the jump size for each parameter in order to obtain a reasonable acceptance rate bounded away from zero and one (see the Appendix for discussion of this point). Overall, the MCMC algorithm mixes quite well for some parameter but less well than others. In the case that $\tau^2 = 0.36$, traceplots from five independent runs of 5000 iterations after 1000 burn-in iterations are given in Figure 4.5. Clearly there is some cause for concern about MCMC error in the computation of posterior quantities, a point we return to shortly.

Table 4.1 reports posterior means and standard deviations of parameters under the $\tau^2 = 0$ and $\tau^2 = 0.36$ scenarios. Given the concern about how well the MCMC algorithm mixes in this example, the table also includes MCMC standard errors reported as a percentage of the computed posterior standard deviation. The MCMC standard error reflects the precision with which a parameter is estimated by the average of estimates from the five independent MCMC runs. It is reported as a percentage of the computed posterior standard deviation, as presumably error arising from the MCMC analysis is only worrisome if it is appreciable relative to the inherent statistical uncertainty about the parameter value. This point is discussed at more length in the Appendix. For most parameters Table 4.1 does indicate that the MCMC error is small relative to statistical uncertainty.

We focus on parameters β_5, β_6, and ω_3^2, as they describe the relationship between the baseline CD4 measurement and the viral dynamics. Table 4.2 gives the posterior mean and standard deviation of each parameter, under all four assumed τ^2 values. We see that the posterior mean of β_6 increases with the assumed value of τ^2. Of course this is to be expected, as a bigger assumed value of τ^2 implies a need for a bigger adjustment to the naive estimate of β_6. Also, the posterior standard deviation of β_6 increases with τ^2, to reflect the larger information loss associated with larger measurement error. Interestingly, the estimated variance of the random effects acting on λ_1 decreases with τ^2.

In comparing the present estimates to those of KD2000, we see that for β_6 both our posterior means and standard deviations tend to be larger than the point estimates and standard errors reported in their paper. Since their approach involves several approximations, we speculate that the present anal-

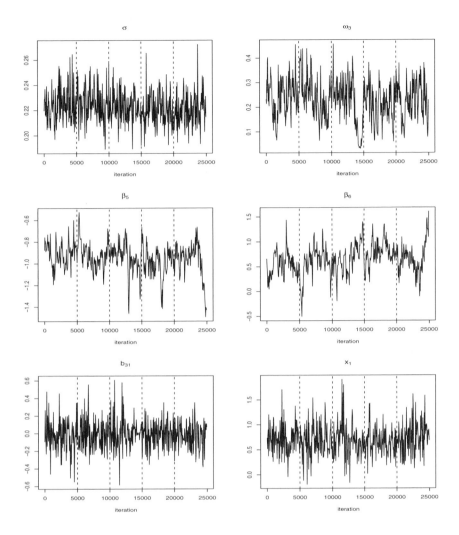

Figure 4.5 *MCMC output for selected quantities in the viral load example of Section 4.3, in the case of $\tau^2 = 0.36$. Output for σ, ω_3, β_5, β_6, b_{31}, and x_1 is given. The dashed horizontal lines separate the output of five independent MCMC runs, each of length 5000. Each run uses 1000 burn-in iterations (not displayed).*

	$\tau^2 = 0$			$\tau^2 = 0.36$		
	Posterior		sim.	Posterior		sim.
	mean	SD	error	mean	SD	error
β_1	12.28	0.15	7%	12.36	0.15	6%
β_2	2.10	0.20	3%	1.76	0.28	8%
β_3	8.12	0.16	14%	8.13	0.16	9%
β_4	1.69	0.20	6%	1.62	0.21	6%
β_5	-0.78	0.08	9%	-0.95	0.14	11%
β_6	0.12	0.10	7%	0.64	0.30	14%
β_7	-3.11	0.10	11%	-3.10	0.09	9%
σ^2	0.05	0.01	2%	0.05	0.01	6%
ω_1^2	0.16	0.12	5%	0.14	0.13	8%
ω_2^2	0.50	0.20	2%	0.52	0.21	6%
ω_3^2	0.10	0.04	2%	0.06	0.04	7%
ω_4^2	0.22	0.08	2%	0.21	0.08	6%
α_0				0.41	0.10	3%
α_1				-0.43	0.15	4%
λ^2				0.12	0.06	6%

Table 4.1 *Parameter estimates in the viral load example under the $\tau^2 = 0$ (no measurement error) and $\tau^2 = 0.36$ scenarios. In each case the posterior mean, posterior standard deviation, and MCMC standard error are given. In particular, the MCMC standard error is reported as a percentage of the posterior standard deviation.*

	$\tau^2 = 0$	$\tau^2 = 0.12$	$\tau^2 = 0.24$	$\tau^2 = 0.36$
$E(\beta_5|\text{data})$	-0.776	-0.801	-0.893	-0.948
$SD(\beta_5|\text{data})$	0.078	0.084	0.113	0.141
$E(\beta_6|\text{data})$	0.122	0.191	0.448	0.642
$SD(\beta_6|\text{data})$	0.089	0.135	0.236	0.287
$E(\omega_3^2|\text{data})$	0.096	0.085	0.084	0.058
$SD(\omega_3^2|\text{data})$	0.038	0.039	0.039	0.038

Table 4.2 *Selected parameter estimates in the viral load example for all four assumed τ^2 values. Posterior means and standard deviations for β_5, β_6, and ω_3^2 are given.*

ysis more fully reflects the various uncertainties at play in arriving at larger uncertainty assessments. This is quite a tentative conclusion, however, given that the MCMC-based estimates are susceptible to simulation error. It would be worthwhile to apply more specialized MCMC algorithms to this problem in an attempt to compute posterior quantities more precisely. Some discussion of more specialized algorithms is given in the Appendix.

4.4 Logistic Regression I: Smoking and Bladder Cancer

The template of measurement model, response model, and exposure model applies equally well to scenarios with a dichotomous response. We illustrate this in the context of a particular medical study, using a subset of the data reported on by Band et $al.$ (1999). These data were collected in an occupational oncology research program, with the aim of identifying cancer risk factors. Relevant information, including cigarette smoking history, was obtained using self-administered questionnaires from 15463 male cancer patients aged 20 years or older. These patients were identified via a population-based cancer registry. In addition to analyzing occupational information, Band et $al.$ also examined the relationship between smoking and cancer for various tumor sites using the case–control approach. For bladder cancer, the cases are the 1038 patients diagnosed with this disease. The controls are those patients diagnosed with other cancers, except those known to be strongly associated with cigarette smoking as described in Wynder and Hoffman (1982). These exceptions include cancers of the lung, lip, oral cavity and pharynx, esophagus, stomach, pancreas, larynx, and kidney. As a result, 7006 controls were identified. The strategy of choosing patients with other cancers, rather than healthy individuals, as controls, has both drawbacks and advantages. It does limit the generalizability of study results. However, in the context of an exposure measured with considerable error it may limit the potential for differential measurement error than can arise in case-control studies. Since the controls and cases are similar in the sense of having a cancer diagnosis, attitudes towards questions about smoking exposure are less likely to vary greatly between the two groups.

The cigarette pack-year, defined as the number of years of smoking twenty cigarettes a day, is used as the exposure variable. For the purposes of illustration we consider only the data on self-reported current or former smokers, i.e., those who report a positive pack-year value on the questionnaire. In doing so we focus on the association between the extent of exposure and disease amongst current and former smokers. This reduction yields $n_0 = 5348$ controls and $n_1 = 914$ cases. For an analysis which includes the non-smokers, see Gustafson, Le and Vallée (2002). In a related vein, we note that Schmid and Rosner (1993) consider measurement and exposure models under which a self-reported zero exposure may or may not correspond to an actual zero exposure. Their work is amongst the first to employ a Bayes-MCMC approach for dealing with mismeasurement.

We consider the response model

$$\text{logit}Pr(Y = 1 | X, Z) \quad = \quad \beta_0 + \beta_1 X + \beta_2 Z, \tag{4.23}$$

where Y is the disease indicator, taking the value zero for controls and one for cases, X is the logarithm of the actual smoking exposure in pack-years, and Z is the patient's age in years. In thinking of such a model we are taking the common approach of analyzing data collected in a *retrospective* case-control study as if they were collected in a *prospective* cohort study. An asymptotic justification for this pretense is given by Prentice and Pyke (1979), although strictly speaking this does not apply to Bayes inference, or to situations involving mismeasured covariates. We will gloss over this point for now, but return to it at length in Section 4.7. In particular, we will introduce a way to check the validity of the pretense in the Bayesian context.

Clearly a self-reported pack-year value will be subject to measurement error. Unfortunately, there is no mechanism by which to rigourously estimate the nature or magnitude of this error. Thus we perform a sensitivity analysis, and draw inferences under different measurement error scenarios. Since the self-reported pack-year value requires a mental assessment of exposure over past years, it is plausible that the magnitude of the measurement error is proportional to the actual exposure. Such multiplicative error on the pack-year scale corresponds to additive error after the logarithmic transform is employed. Letting X^* be the logarithm of the self-reported pack-year value, a simple measurement model would be

$$X^* | Y, X, Z \quad \sim \quad N(X, \tau^2). \tag{4.24}$$

Of course this model assumes the measurement error is nondifferential, unbiased, and normally distributed. More complicated scenarios that relax one or more of these assumptions could be developed; for instance, Gustafson, Le, and Vallée consider scenarios involving a bias, so that $E(X^* | X = x) \neq x$. However, (4.24) is an obvious initial scenario to consider. We try different values of τ in (4.24) to see how inferences vary with the assumed magnitude of the measurement error.

Finally, we require an exposure model. A normal model is convenient. In light of the earlier discussion we require only a model for $X | Z$, rather than (X, Z) jointly. Thus we take

$$X | Z \quad \sim \quad N(\alpha_0 + \alpha_1 Z, \lambda^2).$$

Following the template from Section 4.1, the three component models lead to a posterior distribution of the form

$$f(x, \beta, \alpha, \lambda^2 | x^*, y, z) \quad \propto \quad \prod_{i=1}^{n} \exp\left(-\frac{1}{2}\frac{(x_i^* - x_i)^2}{\tau^2}\right) \times$$

$$\prod_{i=1}^{n} \frac{\exp\{y_i(\beta_0 + \beta_1 x_i + \beta_2 z_i)\}}{1 + \exp(\beta_0 + \beta_1 x_i + \beta_2 z_i)} \times$$

τ	β_1	β_2
0	0.253 (0.039)	0.0177 (0.0031)
0.25	0.267 (0.041)	0.0176 (0.0031)
0.50	0.312 (0.049)	0.0166 (0.0031)

Table 4.3 *Inferences in the smoking and bladder cancer example, under different assumed measurement error magnitudes. The estimates of β_1 and β_2 are posterior means, with posterior standard deviations in parentheses.*

$$\left(\frac{1}{\lambda^2}\right)^{n/2} \prod_{i=1}^{n} \exp\left\{-\frac{1}{2}\frac{(x_i - \alpha_0 - \alpha_1 z_i)^2}{\lambda^2}\right\} \times$$
$$f(\beta, \alpha, \lambda^2). \tag{4.25}$$

We take locally uniform priors for β and α, but use an inverse gamma prior for λ^2. In particular, we again use a unit-information prior for λ^2, with a conservative prior guess taken to be the sample variance of X^*.

While the components of x and β do not have standard full conditional distributions, MCMC simulation from the posterior distribution given by (4.25) is still relatively straightforward. Some implementation details are given in Section 4.11. Posterior means and standard deviations for the coefficients β_1 and β_2 appear in Table 4.3, assuming $\tau = 0$, $\tau = 0.25$, and $\tau = 0.5$ respectively. Referring back to the original pack-year exposure scale, these values can be regarded as corresponding to no measurement error, 25% multiplicative error, and 50% multiplicative error respectively. Qualitatively, inferences about the exposure coefficient β_1 behave as expected. The posterior mean of β_1 increases with the assumed value of τ, to compensate for a bigger assumed attenuation. Also, the posterior standard deviation of β_1 increases with τ, to reflect less information about the actual exposures. Note, however, that the increase in the estimate of β_1 under $\tau = 0.25$ relative to $\tau = 0$ is quite slight. Moreover, even when $\tau = 0.5$ the posterior mean of β_1 is only one posterior standard deviation larger than the posterior mean when $\tau = 0$. Finally, the posterior mean of β_2 is quite insensitive to the assumed value of τ. In light of the results in Chapter 2, this suggests that X and Z are not strongly correlated. Indeed, the sample correlation between X^* and Z is only 0.16.

Overall, since $\tau = 0$ to $\tau = 0.5$ spans a range from no measurement error to a very substantial multiplicative measurement error in pack-year exposure, we have some confidence that inferences arrived at assuming no measurement error are not badly biased by the measurement error. This is comforting in the face of an exposure such as smoking where this is little hope of ascertaining the precise magnitude of the measurement error via gold-standard measurements, replicated measurements, or other techniques.

4.5 Logistic Regression II: Framingham Heart Study

As a second example of incorporating measurement error with a binary out-come variable, we consider data from an epidemiological cohort study. The Framingham Heart study involves a large cohort followed over a long period of time (Dawber, Kannel and Lyell 1963). We consider the data accrued from the initial exam through the first ten biennial follow-up exams, taking the outcome variable to be twenty-year mortality from any cause. Explanatory variables, as recorded on initial exam, include age, gender, weight, smoking status, serum cholesterol level, diastolic blood pressure, and systolic blood pressure. Given the choice of twenty-year mortality as the outcome variable, we restrict attention to the subset of the cohort aged 55 or younger at the initial exam, yielding a sample of size $n = 4526$.

Several of the explanatory variables are measured with error. We focus on serum cholesterol, for which measurements at both the initial exam and the first follow-up exam are available, at least for the majority of subjects. The 'true' level of serum cholesterol is assumed constant across the initial and first follow-up exams, with the two measurements taken as pure replicates. Also, examination of the measured values suggests that a normality assumption is more appropriate for the logarithm of the measurements. Thus if X represents the logarithm of the true serum cholesterol level (in mg/100ml), while X_1^* and X_2^* are the logarithms of the measured values at the initial and first follow-up exams respectively, we entertain the nondifferential measurement model

$$\begin{pmatrix} X_1^* \\ X_2^* \end{pmatrix} | X, Z, Y \Big) \sim N\left\{ \begin{pmatrix} X \\ X \end{pmatrix}, \begin{pmatrix} \tau^2 & 0 \\ 0 & \tau^2 \end{pmatrix} \right\}.$$

Here Y is the response variable (coded as zero/one for alive/dead twenty years after initial exam), while Z is a vector of other explanatory variables. In line with the previous examples, the response and conditional exposure models are taken to be

$$logit\{Pr(Y = 1|X, Z)\} = \beta_0 + \beta_1 X + \beta_2' Z,$$

and

$$X|Z \sim N(\alpha_0 + \alpha_1' Z, \lambda^2).$$

The precisely measured explanatory variables Z include both linear and quadratic terms for age at initial exam, specifically $(AGE - 42)$ and $(AGE - 42)^2$, where 42 is the average initial age in the sub-cohort being considered. Clearly age at initial exam will be a very important predictor in a twenty-year mortality study, so both linear and quadratic terms are included in an attempt to fully account for this explanatory variable. Other components of Z include gender (coded as zero/one for male/female), smoking status at initial exam (coded as zero/one for no/yes), 'metropolitan relative weight' at initial exam (coded as percentage of 'normal'), diastolic blood pressure as measured at initial exam (in mm-Hg), and systolic blood pressure as measured at initial exam (in mm-Hg).

	$\hat{\beta}$	(PSD)	$\exp\left(\hat{\beta}\right)$
AGE_1	0.083	(0.008)	1.09
AGE_2	-0.001	(0.001)	1.00
GENDER	-0.475	(0.091)	0.62
SMOKING	0.756	(0.095)	2.13
LOG-CHOL	0.131	(0.120)	1.14
RELWHT	-0.009	(0.046)	0.99
DBP	0.140	(0.071)	1.15
SBP	0.316	(0.068)	1.37

Table 4.4 *Estimated coefficients in the Framingham analysis. For each coefficient the estimate $\hat{\beta}$ is the posterior mean, with the posterior standard deviation (PSD) given in parentheses. The corresponding adjusted odds-ratio $\exp\left(\hat{\beta}\right)$ is also given. The AGE_1 and AGE_2 coefficients are reported as log odds-ratios with respect to $(age-42)$ and $(age-42)^2$. The $LOG-CHOL$ coefficient is reported with respect to a change of $\log(1.5)$ in log serum-cholesterol; hence the odds-ratio can be interpreted in relation to a 50% increase in the serum-cholesterol level. Each of the RELWHT, DBP, and SBP coefficients are reported with respect to a one standard-deviation change in the explanatory variable.*

The approach to prior construction and MCMC fitting used in the previous example (and discussed in Section 4.11) is easily adapted to the present setting. We again employ locally uniform prior distributions for the response model coefficients β and the conditional exposure model coefficients α, and unit-information inverse gamma priors for τ^2 and λ^2. To be conservative, the prior guesses for both τ^2 and λ^2 are taken to be the sample variance of X_1^*. One twist in the present scenario is that one or both X^* measurements are missing for some subjects. It is easy to see, however, that the conditional distribution of say X_{1i}^* given all other quantities is simply given by the measurement model as $N(X_i, \tau^2)$. Thus it is trivial to extend the MCMC algorithm to also update the missing values of X^*.

Examination of a posterior sample of size 5000 reveals fast convergence and good mixing. This output yields the posterior means and standard deviations for the components of β which appear in Table 4.4. Note that the LOG-CHOL coefficient β_1 is reported with respect to a change of $\log(1.5)$ units on the log-cholesterol scale, so that the corresponding odds-ratio can be interpreted with respect to a 50% increase in cholesterol level. Note also that the posterior mean of τ is 0.10, which is quite large in relation to the sample standard deviations of $SD(X_1^*) = 0.2$ and $SD(X_2^*) = 0.19$. Thus the data suggest substantial measurement error is manifested.

By way of contrast, an analogous analysis which ignores measurement error is also considered. This analysis treats the first cholesterol measurement as exact when it is available, and substitutes the second measurement for the first in the 1686 cases where the first is missing but the second is not. The 107 subjects with both measurements missing are omitted. Again parameterized relative to an additive change of log(1.5) in log-cholesterol, a posterior mean and standard deviation of 0.120 and 0.093 are obtained for the corresponding logistic regression coefficient. In particular, these values are obtained from direct MCMC fitting of the outcome model only, with observed X values. Relative to this naive analysis then, adjusting for measurement error leads to both a bigger estimated coefficient and a larger assessment of statistical uncertainty about the coefficient. The changes are relatively slight in both cases, however, despite indications of substantial measurement error. The MCMC output also yields the posterior probability that the log-cholesterol coefficient is positive given the data. Specifically, this is computed to be 0.86 in the model which adjusts for measurement error and 0.89 in the model which does not. Thus the adjustment does *not* lead to stronger evidence of a cholesterol effect on mortality, since the modest increase in the estimated coefficient is in fact more than offset by the modest increase in the posterior standard deviation of the coefficient.

4.6 Issues in Specifying the Exposure Model

A common criticism of the parametric approach to measurement error problems is that one runs the risk of specifying a distributional form for the exposure distribution that is far from correct. Of course this can be construed as a criticism of all parametric statistical modelling, though one might argue that the problem is particularly acute for exposure models. In particular, it is hard to check empirically whether a postulated exposure model seems reasonable, simply because the exposure variable itself is not observed. Some advocate trying to avoid the specification of an exposure model all together. We will comment on such methods in Section 4.9. Others advocate the use of very flexible models for exposure distributions. For instance, in a non-Bayesian context Roeder, Carroll and Lindsay (1996) use semiparametric mixture modelling for the exposure distribution. In the Bayesian context Muller and Roeder (1997), Carroll, Roeder and Wasserman (1999), and Richardson, Leblond, Jaussent and Green (2002) use mixture models for the exposure distribution, while Mallick, Hoffman and Carroll (2002) consider a different approach based on the Pólya tree prior (Lavine 1992).

Notwithstanding these approaches, typically the inferential focus is on parameters in the response model, which is one level removed from the exposure model. Intuitively one might imagine that this separation would act as a buffer, so that a considerable misspecification of the exposure distribution might yield only a mild bias in estimators of the response model parameters. Indeed, the emphasis in the literature on misspecification at the level of exposure model seems slightly odd, as one might imagine that misspecification of the measurement model, or of the response model itself, would be a bigger problem in practice. This point is returned to later in Section 6.2.

As an initial investigation of the role of the exposure model, consider the normal model discussed in Section 4.2, in the further restricted scenario that τ^2 is known (say from previous studies) and only a single X^* measurement is made for each subject. Thus a joint distribution for $(X^*, Y, X|Z)$ is assumed to be of the form

$$
\begin{aligned}
X^*|Y, X, Z &\sim N\left(X, \tau^2\right), \\
Y|X, Z &\sim N\left(\beta_0 + \beta_1 X + \beta_2 Z, \sigma^2\right), \\
X|Z &\sim N\left(\alpha_0 + \alpha_1 Z, \lambda^2\right),
\end{aligned}
$$

with a total of seven unknown parameters. As discussed in Section 4.2, this implies a collapsed model for $(Y, X^*|Z)$ with the normal forms (4.9) for $(Y|X^*, Z)$ and (4.10) for $(X^*|Z)$. In particular, the one-to-one mapping between the initial parameterization $\theta = (\beta_0, \beta_1, \beta_2, \alpha_0, \alpha_1, \sigma^2, \lambda^2)$ and the parameterization of the collapsed model $\tilde{\theta} = (\tilde{\beta}_0, \tilde{\beta}_1, \tilde{\beta}_2, \tilde{\alpha}_0, \tilde{\alpha}_1, \tilde{\sigma}^2, \tilde{\lambda}^2)$ is given by (4.11) through (4.17). We focus on inference about β_1 in the outcome model, which can be expressed in terms of collapsed model parameters as

$$
\beta_1 = \left(1 + \frac{\tau^2}{\tilde{\lambda}^2 - \tau^2}\right)\tilde{\beta}_1. \tag{4.26}
$$

In studying the large-sample behaviour of estimators we write $AVAR$ to denote the asymptotic variance of an estimator and $ACOV$ to denote the asymptotic covariance between two estimators. That is, for consistent estimators $(\hat{\psi}_1, \hat{\psi}_2)$ of parameters (ψ_1, ψ_2)

$$
n^{1/2}\left(\begin{array}{cc} AVAR[\psi_1] & ACOV[\psi_1, \psi_2] \\ ACOV[\psi_1, \psi_2] & AVAR[\psi_2] \end{array}\right)^{-1/2}\left(\begin{array}{c} \hat{\psi}_1 - \psi_1 \\ \hat{\psi}_2 - \psi_2 \end{array}\right) \Rightarrow N_2\left(0, I\right),
$$

where $N_2(0, I)$ denotes the bivariate standard normal distribution, and the convergence is in distribution, as the sample size n tends to infinity.

We can express the asymptotic variance incurred in estimating β_1 in terms of asymptotic variances and covariances in the collapsed model, using the well-known 'Delta method' based on a Taylor series expansion. Applied to (4.26) it yields

$$
\begin{aligned}
AVAR\left[\beta_1\right] = {} & \left(1 + \frac{\tau^2}{\tilde{\lambda}^2 - \tau^2}\right)^2 AVAR\left[\tilde{\beta}_1\right] + \\
& \left\{\frac{\tau^4 \tilde{\beta}_1^2}{(\tilde{\lambda}^2 - \tau^2)^4}\right\} AVAR\left[\tilde{\lambda}^2\right] + \\
& \left\{\frac{-2\tilde{\lambda}^2 \tau^2 \tilde{\beta}_1}{(\tilde{\lambda}^2 - \tau^2)^3}\right\} ACOV\left[\tilde{\beta}_1, \tilde{\lambda}^2\right]. \tag{4.27}
\end{aligned}
$$

Now the readily computed Fisher information matrix for the collapsed model gives

$$
\begin{aligned}
AVAR\left[\tilde{\beta}_1\right] &= \tilde{\sigma}^2/\tilde{\lambda}^2, \\
AVAR\left[\tilde{\lambda}^2\right] &= 2\tilde{\lambda}^4, \\
ACOV\left[\tilde{\beta}_1, \tilde{\lambda}^2\right] &= 0.
\end{aligned}
$$

Plugging these expressions into (4.27), and expressing the result in terms of the original parameterization, gives

$$AVAR[\beta_1] \quad = \quad \frac{\sigma^2}{\lambda^2}\left(1 + \frac{1}{1-\rho^2}\Delta + \frac{2\rho^2}{1-\rho^2}\Delta^2\right), \tag{4.28}$$

where $\Delta = \tau^2/\lambda^2 = Var(X^*|X,Z)/Var(X|Z)$ is the measurement error magnitude expressed as a proportion of the conditional variance of X given Z, while $\rho^2 = \{Cor(Y,X|Z)\}^2 = \beta_1^2\lambda^2/(\sigma^2 + \beta_1^2\lambda^2)$ indicates the strength of the relationship between X and Y given Z. Note that (4.28) increases with Δ, to reflect the loss of information incurred as the magnitude of the measurement error increases.

Hypothetically, if the parameters of the exposure model were known rather than estimated, then the asymptotic variance of $\hat{\beta}_1$ would be given by only the first of the three terms in (4.27), and consequently by only the first two of the three terms in (4.28). That is, the proportion of $AVAR\left[\hat{\beta}_1\right]$ due to uncertainty about the exposure model depends only on Δ and ρ, and can be expressed as

$$w(\Delta, \rho) \quad = \quad \frac{2\rho^2\Delta^2}{1 - \rho^2 + \Delta + 2\rho^2\Delta^2}. \tag{4.29}$$

This proportion is plotted as a function of Δ in Figure 4.6, for some specific values of ρ. We see that unless the outcome-exposure relationship is very strong (ρ large), or the measurement error is quite large (Δ large), inference about β_1 is *not* substantially improved by knowing the correct parameter values in the exposure model. This provides a sense in which the exposure model is not particularly influential in the estimation of an outcome model parameter.

Given that in many circumstances the exposure model seems not to contribute very much to inferences about the outcome model parameters, one might posit that using an incorrect exposure model will not be terribly damaging. In fact, in situations where the measurement, response, and exposure models are all normal linear models, estimators of the response model parameters are remarkably robust in the face of an actual exposure distribution which differs from the postulated exposure model. Quite general results along these lines are given by Fuller (1987). To shed light on this we present two results which are proved in Section 4.11.

Result 4.1 *Assume that (Y, X, Z) jointly have finite second moments, and say X^* and (Y, Z) are conditionally independent given X, with $E(X^*|X) = X$, and $Var(X^*|X) = \tau^2$, where τ^2 is known. Let l_0 be the large-sample limit of the X coefficient from a linear regression of Y on $(1, X, Z)$, with independent realizations of (Y, X, Z). Now consider fitting the model which assumes (i) $X^*|Y, X, Z \sim N(X, \tau^2)$, (ii) $Y|X, Z \sim N(\beta_0 + \beta_1 X + \beta_2 Z, \sigma^2)$, and (iii) $X|Z \sim N(\alpha_0 + \alpha_1 Z, \lambda^2)$, to independent realizations of (Y, X^*, Z). Let l_1 be the large-sample limit of a Bayes or maximum likelihood estimator of β_1. This estimator is consistent, in the sense that $l_1 = l_0$.*

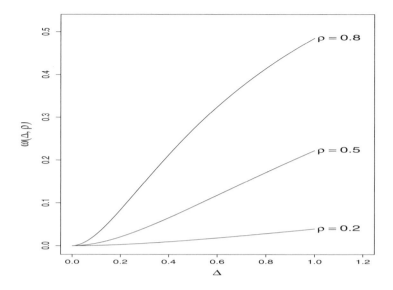

Figure 4.6 *Proportion of $AVAR[\beta_1]$ due to uncertainty about the exposure model parameters. Specifically, $w(\Delta, \rho)$ defined by (4.29) is plotted as a function of $\Delta = Var(X^*|X)/Var(X)$, for selected values of $\rho = Cor(X, Y|Z)$.*

We emphasize that here nothing is being assumed about the correctness or incorrectness of the response model, as was also stressed in many of the Chapter 2 results. Also, the measurement model is only assumed to be correct up to first and second moments. Thus the result is somewhat more general than that given by Fuller (1987). The important content of the result is that regardless of the real shape of the exposure distribution, the postulated normal linear exposure distribution will suffice to give the same limiting estimate as would be obtained by applying the response model alone to (Y, X, Z) data. Put succinctly, incorrectly postulating a normal linear exposure model does not induce any asymptotic bias in the estimation of β_1.

While this robustness to exposure model misspecification in the sense of consistency may seem somewhat remarkable in its own right, in fact an even stronger statement obtains. Specifically, the asymptotic variance of the estimator is unaffected by the extent to which the exposure model is misspecified. For simplicity we give this result in the simpler context of no additional precisely measured covariates. Fuller (1987) gives such a result in a more general context.

Result 4.2 *Consider a Bayesian or maximum likelihood estimator $\hat{\beta}_1$ of β_1 based on fitting three-part model (i) $X^*|Y, X \sim N(X, \tau^2)$, (ii) $Y|X \sim N(\beta_0 + \beta_1 X, \sigma^2)$, and (iii) $X \sim N(\alpha_0, \lambda^2)$, to n independent realizations of (X^*, Y). Here τ^2 is known, while $(\beta_1, \beta_1, \alpha_0, \sigma^2, \lambda^2)$ are unknown. Now say that in fact (i) and (ii) are correct specifications, so that we can write β_0, β_1, and σ^2*

unambiguously as 'true' parameter values. Also say that X has an arbitrary distribution with finite variance. Of course Result 4.1 implies that $\hat{\beta}_1$ is a consistent estimator of β_1. But now the asymptotic variance of $\hat{\beta}_1$ is given by

$$AVAR[\beta_1] \quad = \quad \frac{\sigma^2}{Var(X)}\left(1 + \frac{1}{1-\rho^2}\Delta + \frac{2\rho^2}{1-\rho^2}\Delta^2\right), \qquad (4.30)$$

where

$$\begin{aligned}
\rho \quad &= \quad Cor(Y, X) \\
&= \quad \frac{\beta_1}{\{\sigma^2 + \beta_1^2 Var(X)\}^{1/2}},
\end{aligned}$$

and $\Delta = \tau^2/Var(X)$ is the measurement error variance expressed as a proportion of $Var(X)$. In particular, the asymptotic variance of the estimator depends only on the variance of X, not on the shape of distribution. Thus the asymptotic distribution of the estimator is entirely unaffected by the extent to which the true exposure distribution does or does not match the postulated normal distribution.

We note in passing that (4.30) matches (4.28) in the case that an additional precisely measured covariate is involved. Taken together, Results 4.1 and 4.2 support the use of a normal exposure model regardless of whether this is viewed as plausible in the scenario at hand.

It is folklore in statistical science that phenomena arising in normal linear models tend to be approximately manifested in generalized linear models as well. Thus the extreme insensitivity to exposure distribution misspecification arising with normal response models might be expected to carry over to binary response models. Some recent work, however, speaks against this to some extent. Richardson and Leblond (1997) consider normal linear measurement and exposure models in conjunction with a logistic regression model for the binary outcome Y given imprecisely measured exposure variable X and precisely measured covariate Z. They apply Bayes-MCMC fitting to simulated data, and demonstrate some deterioration in the estimation of response model coefficients as the true exposure distribution deviates from a normal distribution. They summarize their findings as having shown "some sensitivity to misspecification, the overall picture being that of a moderate bias in the estimates and increased posterior standard deviations." We note in passing that Richardson and Leblond consider an exposure model for X alone, while the outcome model is for Y given both X and Z. This is tantamount to assuming that X and Z are independent of one another, so that the requisite conditional exposure model for $X|Z$ can be reduced to a model for X alone. However, they explicitly simulate datasets which involve positive correlation between X and Z. Thus there is a second aspect to the misspecification that is not acknowledged by the authors—both the shape of the postulated X distribution and the postulated independence of X and Z are violated in their simulated scenarios.

In their investigation of mixture modelling for the exposure distribution,

Richardson, Leblond, Jaussent and Green (2002) also make reference to the use of misspecified exposure models. The scenario is that of a nondifferential normal measurement model for $X^*|X$, a logistic regression model for $Y|X$, and a mixture-of-normals model for X. Additional precisely measured covariates are not considered. The exposure model is quite flexible, as the number of components in the mixture, the weight of each component, and the mean and variance of each component are all treated as unknown parameters. Reversible jump MCMC (Green 1995) is used to deal with the varying dimensional parameter space, as exemplified for mixtures by Richardson and Green (1997). On simulated data, Richardson, Leblond, Jaussent and Green compare estimates arising under their flexible exposure model to those arising from a simple normal exposure model. For several scenarios where the true exposure distribution is grossly nonnormal, they report mean-squared errors for outcome model coefficients that are considerably larger under the normal exposure model than under the flexible exposure model. In light of these findings it seems relevant to consider more flexible exposure models.

4.7 More Flexible Exposure Models

Some Bayesian approaches to flexible exposure models in tandem with non-normal response models have been considered recently in the literature. Much of this work involves mixture models, as in Carroll, Roeder and Wasserman (1999), Muller and Roeder (1997), and Richardson, Leblond, Jaussent and Green (2002). The approach of Roeder, Carroll and Lindsay (1996), while not Bayesian, pursues a similar tack.

Some of the suggested techniques for flexible exposure distribution modelling are quite demanding to implement and execute. Gustafson, Le and Vallée (2002) suggest the arguably simpler approach of modelling the exposure distribution as a discrete distribution on a suitably large set of support points. To illustrate this in a simple context, say there is a single imprecisely measured exposure variable with no additional precisely measured covariates. Let $f_M(x^*|x, y)$ be the completely known measurement model and let $f_R(y|x, \theta_R)$ be the response model. Let $g[1] < g[2] < \ldots < g[m-1] < g[m]$ denote the m fixed support points of the exposure distribution for X. It is convenient to introduce an indexing variable $a_i \in \{1, \ldots, m\}$ for each subject, such that $x_i = g[a_i]$. Then $a = (a_1, \ldots, a_n)$ rather than $x = (x_1, \ldots, x_n)$ can be viewed as describing the unobserved exposures. In particular, an exposure model parameterized by θ_E is specified as $f_E(a|\theta_E)$, giving the joint posterior density of interest as

$$
\begin{aligned}
f(a, \theta_R, \theta_E | x^*, y) \quad &\propto \quad \prod_{i=1}^{n} f_M(x_i^*|g[a_i], y_i) f_R(y_i|g[a_i], \theta_R) \; \times \\
&\quad \prod_{i=1}^{n} f_E(a_i|\theta_E) \; \times \\
&\quad f(\theta_R, \theta_E).
\end{aligned}
\tag{4.31}
$$

In fact the obvious exposure model simply assigns a probability to each gridpoint, which we express as $Pr(a_i = j|\gamma) = \gamma_j$. Put more succinctly, $a_1, \ldots, a_n$ are modelled as independent and identically distributed from the Multinomial$(1, \gamma)$ distribution, where $\gamma = (\gamma_1, \ldots, \gamma_m)$. A simple noninformative prior for γ would be a uniform distribution over the m-dimensional probability simplex, which is equivalently the Dirichlet$(1, \ldots, 1)$ distribution. Since the Dirichlet distribution is a conjugate prior for a Multinomial model, MCMC updating of γ is easily accomplished via Gibbs sampling. More specifically, the joint posterior density (4.31) specializes to

$$
f(a, \theta_R, \gamma | x^*, y) \propto \prod_{i=1}^{n} f_M(x_i^* | g[a_i], y_i) f_R(y_i | g[a_i], \theta_R) \times
$$

$$
\prod_{j=1}^{m} \gamma_j^{c_j(a)} \times
$$

$$
f(\theta_R), \tag{4.32}
$$

where $c_j(a) = \sum_{i=1}^{n} I\{a_i = j\}$ is the number of x values currently assigned to the j-th support point. In terms of MCMC updating, whatever strategy might be used to update θ_R under a parametric exposure model can be used here without modification. Moreover, as mentioned above, updating γ is straightforward. The remaining issue is how to update the components of a. A simple approach is to use a discrete version of the random walk MH algorithm.

That is, candidates of the form $a_i^* = a_i + V$ are generated, where V is a symmetric distribution on $\{-k, \ldots, -1, 1, \ldots, k\}$ for a suitably chosen value of k. As a minor point, care must be taken at either end of the grid, perhaps by using 'reflection' to maintain candidate moves for which the reverse moves are equally likely. That is, the precise candidate generation scheme is

$$
a_i^* = \begin{cases} 1 + \{(1 - (a_i + V)\} & \text{if } a_i + V < 1, \\ m - \{(a_i + V) - m\} & \text{if } a_i + V > m, \\ a_i + V & \text{otherwise.} \end{cases}
$$

Then the MH algorithm acceptance probability is based simply on the ratio of (4.32) at the candidate value to (4.32) at the current value. Since (4.32) factors into separate terms for each a_i, these updates can be carried out efficiently in a parallel fashion.

As noted by Gustafson, Le and Vallée (2002), there are competing desiderata in selecting the fixed support points for the exposure distribution. Say the measurement model is simply $X^* | Y, X \sim N(X, \tau^2)$ where τ^2 is known, as would be the case in a sensitivity analysis, for instance. On the one hand, we want the number of support points m to be small, relative to the sample size n in particular. This is needed if one hopes to estimate the probabilities γ well. On the other hand, the spacing of the grid points cannot be too large in relation to τ if one wants the discrete approximation to the distribution of X given X^* and parameters to be faithful to the underlying 'true' smooth distribution. Viewing the second desideratum as more pressing than the first, we choose an equally-spaced grid, with $g[1] = min_i\{x_i^*\} - 2.5\tau$, $g[m] = max_i\{x_i^*\} + 2.5\tau$, and a spacing between adjacent gridpoints of $\tau/4$. This spacing can be viewed as giving a 16-point approximation to the main body $(x \pm 2\tau)$ of the conditional distribution for $X^*|X = x$ viewed as a function of x. Of course the method is expected to perform better when the resulting m is small compared to the sample size n. In turn, this suggests better performance when τ is larger. Gustafson, Le and Vallée (2002) suggest using the same choice of gridpoints based on an estimated value of τ in validation designs where X is observed for some subjects and τ is not known in advance. In general, grid-based statistical models are often unattractive because it is unclear how to choose the coarseness of the grid. In measurement error models, however, either complete or rough knowledge of the measurement error magnitude provides guidance for the choice of grid spacing.

Of course most studies do involve additional precisely measured covariates, so the exposure model requires a conditional distribution for $(X|Z)$ rather than a marginal distribution for X. It is a formidable challenge to construct flexible models for a conditional distribution of X given p other covariates Z. Indeed, none of the mixture model based approaches mentioned earlier have been extended to this more general scenario. Similarly, direct adaptation of the grid approach above would require each probability γ_j to be a function of Z. To avoid such a complicated structure, Gustafson, Le and Vallée (2002) resort to assuming that X and Z are independent. Clearly such an assumption is grossly violated in many applications.

A middle ground approach is to use what we term a *reverse-exposure* model, which postulates a joint distribution for (X, Z) in terms of the grid-based model for the marginal distribution of X along with a simple parametric model for Z given X. Of course this is literally a 'reverse' situation, as we have already illustrated that generally if a model for $X|Z$ is postulated then it is not necessary to postulate a model for Z. But particularly in situations where the association between X and Z is not suspected to be strong, the overall effect of using a very flexible model for X and a parametric model for $Z|X$ will be a reasonably flexible model for $X|Z$.

In particular, with a parametric model $f_{RE}(z|x, \theta_{RE})$ for $Z|X$ (RE standing for Reverse Exposure), the posterior density (4.32) generalizes to

$$
\begin{aligned}
f(a, \theta_R, \theta_{RE}, \gamma | x^*, y) \quad &\propto \quad \prod_{i=1}^{n} f_M(x_i^* | g[a_i], y_i) f_R(y_i | g[a_i], \theta_R) \; \times \\
&\prod_{j=1}^{m} \gamma_j^{c_j(a)} \; \times \\
&\prod_{i=1}^{n} f_{RE}(z_i | g[a_i], \theta_{RE}) \; \times \\
&f(\theta_R, \theta_{RE}). \qquad\qquad\qquad (4.33)
\end{aligned}
$$

Note that MCMC fitting is only slightly more complicated when using (4.33) as opposed to (4.32). The updating of θ_R remains unchanged, as does the Dirichlet updating of γ. The discretized random-walk MH algorithm can again be used to update a, with the only extension being the need to include the f_{RE} terms in the calculation of acceptance probabilities. Finally, updating of θ_{RE} would typically be straightforward, based on the observed z values and the current x values implied by the current a values.

We try the grid-based reverse exposure model for the smoking and bladder cancer example of Section 4.4. Recall that this example involves log pack-years as the X variable and age as the Z variable. The normal linear exposure model for $X|Z$ is replaced by the grid model for X and a normal linear model for $Z|X$. Note that the selection of gridpoints outlined above leads to $m = 155$ gridpoints when $\tau = 0.25$, and $m = 88$ gridpoints when $\tau = 0.5$. Given the sample size is $n = 6262$, we do have scenarios where m/n is small, as desired.

The MCMC mixing of the outcome model parameters seems comparable to that observed with the simpler model of Section 4.4. The resulting posterior means of $\hat{\beta}_1 = 0.270$ in the $\tau = 0.25$ scenario and $\hat{\beta}_1 = 0.315$ in the $\tau = 0.5$ scenario are essentially indistinguishable from those given in Table 4.3 for the normal exposure model, particularly in light of the posterior standard deviations reported there. In fact, breaking the present MCMC output of 5000 iterations into ten batches of size 500 yields simulation standard errors of 0.002 when $\tau = 0.25$ and 0.003 when $\tau = 0.5$, so that the present posterior means are within 'numerical tolerance' of those arising from the simpler exposure model. In the present example, then, there is no apparent effect of moving to a more flexible exposure model. Of course it is always comforting when inferences are essentially unchanged upon moving to a more flexible model.

It is interesting to examine the estimated exposure distribution that arises from fitting the grid-based reverse exposure model. In particular, the posterior mean of γ corresponds to the estimated distribution of X displayed in the middle panels of Figure 4.7, for $\tau = 0.25$ and $\tau = 0.5$ respectively. While there is some roughness, as one might expect from a grid-based model, there is also a clear suggestion of nonnormality in the sense of a long left tail. As a check on the plausibility of the estimated X distribution, replicated X^* distributions are created. That is a sample of n replicated X^* values is created by first sampling X values from the estimated discrete distribution of X, and then adding $N(0, \tau^2)$ noise to these values. Histograms of these replicated X^* samples appear in the bottom panels of Figure 4.7, using the gridpoints as midpoints of the histogram bins. These can then be compared to the histograms of the actual X^* values in the top panels of Figure 4.7. Generally the actual and replicated X^* samples are quite similar, suggesting the procedure has done a reasonable job of estimating the X distribution. Of course, even though the estimated X distribution is decidedly nonnormal, it still yields estimates of the response model parameters that are essentially the same as those arising from a normal model for the X distribution.

In general it seems that consideration of when flexible exposure models are needed and how best to achieve such flexibility are ripe areas for further research. In the case of logistic-regression response models, the lack of applicable asymptotics means the evidence on how well misspecified normal exposure models work in estimating response model parameters is quite limited. As mentioned, Richardson and Leblond (1997) and Richardson, Leblond, Jaussent and Green (2002) do provide some evidence in favour of using more complex models. Conversely, in the example above a more flexible model provides evidence of a nonnormal exposure distribution, yet estimates of the response model parameter are essentially the same as under a normal exposure model. In light of these findings, further investigation is warranted. A second avenue for investigation involves the comparison of Bayesian methods allowing a flexible exposure model to non-Bayesian counterparts. Outwardly it seems that a flexible exposure model is more easily accommodated within the Bayesian paradigm, but careful comparisons have not been drawn.

4.8 Retrospective Analysis

We now return to a point which was glossed over earlier in this chapter. In Section 4.4 we analyzed the retrospectively collected data on smoking and bladder cancer as if it were collected prospectively. This is common practice in biostatistics, based primarily on a justification given by Prentice and Pyke (1979). This work, however, does not apply to Bayesian analysis, nor to situations involving measurement error. This point has received recent attention from Roeder, Carroll and Lindsay (1996), Muller and Roeder (1997), Seaman and Richardson (2001), and Gustafson, Le and Vallée (2002).

One possibility for analyzing retrospectively collected data subject to measurement error is to use simple parametric models for the distribution of explanatory variables given the outcome variable. This approach has received attention from Armstrong, Whittemore and Howe (1989), Buonaccorsi (1990), and also Gustafson, Le and Vallée (2000) in a Bayesian context. There is some concern, however, that these methods will be particularly lacking in robustness to model misspecification.

Gustafson, Le and Vallée (2002) consider Bayesian modelling which formally accounts for the retrospective way in which the data are collected, while taking advantage of the simpler posterior distribution arising under a prospective model. In particular, they present a scheme to represent the posterior distribution arising from retrospective analysis by reweighting a Monte Carlo sample from the posterior distribution based on prospective data collection. For simplicity we review this approach in the context of a single mismeasured predictor without additional precisely measured covariates.

Say that in the population of interest the prospective relationship between outcome Y and predictor X is governed by a logistic regression model

$$\text{logit} Pr(Y = 1|X) = \tilde{\beta}_0 + \beta_1 X.$$

The fundamental link between this prospective relationship for Y given X and the retrospective relationship for X given Y is succinctly expressed as

$$\log \frac{f(x|y=1)}{f(x|y=0)} = \text{logit}\{Pr(Y=1|X=x)\} - \text{logit}\{Pr(Y=1)\}$$

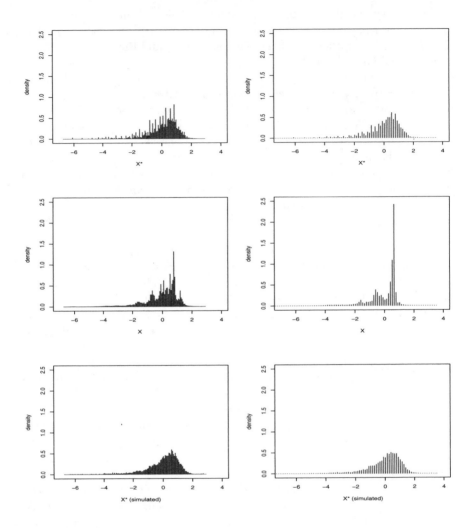

Figure 4.7 *Actual distribution of X^* and estimated distribution of X in the example of Section 4.7. The left panels correspond to assumed measurement error of magnitude $\tau = 0.25$, while the right panels correspond to $\tau = 0.5$. In either case the gridpoint spacing is $\tau/4$. The top panels give histograms of the observed (and centred) X^* with respect to the grid spacing. The middle panels give the estimated distribution of X corresponding to the posterior mean of γ. The bottom panels give histograms of a 'replicated' sample of X^* obtained by adding simulated measurement error to a sample from the estimated distribution of X.*

$$= \quad \beta_0^* + \beta_1 x, \tag{4.34}$$

where

$$\beta_0^* \quad = \quad \tilde{\beta}_0 - \text{logit}\{Pr(Y = 1)\}. \tag{4.35}$$

Note that (4.35) underscores the well-known fact that the prospective intercept $\tilde{\beta}_0$ cannot be estimated from retrospective data without knowledge of the outcome prevalence $Pr(Y = 1)$.

One approach is to assume $f(x|y = 0)$ belongs to some parametric family indexed by ω. Then (β_1, ω) would completely parameterize the problem, as β_0^* would be a deterministic function of (β_1, ω) in order to ensure that

$$f(x|y = 1) \quad = \quad \exp(\beta_0^* + \beta_1 x) f(x|y = 0)$$

is a normalized density function. However, to mimic the role of an exposure model, it is useful to instead assume that

$$h(x) = r f(x|y = 0) + (1 - r) f(x|y = 1) \tag{4.36}$$

belongs to some parametric family of densities indexed by ω. In particular, we fix $r = n_0/(n_0 + n_1)$. Then the case-control sampling scheme can be thought of as first selecting at random $Y = 0$ with probability r or $Y = 1$ with probability $1 - r$, and then sampling X given Y. Under such a sampling scheme (4.36) is the marginal distribution of X, and thereby is akin to the exposure distribution. Thus we henceforth refer to (4.36) as the *pseudo-exposure* distribution.

If we do take $h(x) = h(x|\omega)$ to belong to a parametric family of densities indexed by ω, then the density of X given Y is parameterized by (β_1, ω) according to

$$f(x|y) \quad = \quad \frac{\exp\{y(\beta_0^* + \beta_1 x)\}}{r + (1 - r)\exp(\beta_0^* + \beta_1 x)} \, h(x|\omega).$$

Here β_0^* is a deterministic function of (β_1, ω) given as the solution to

$$E_\omega \left\{ \frac{1}{\beta_0^* + \beta_1 X} \right\} \quad = \quad 1,$$

where the expectation is with respect to X having density $h(\cdot|\omega)$.

Now say that X^* is observed as a surrogate for X, with a completely specified nondifferential measurement model. That is, $X^*|X, Y \equiv X^*|X$ has a known distribution. The retrospective data collection then implies a posterior distribution for the unknown values of X along with the unknown parameters (β_1^*, ω) as

$$f(x, \beta_1, \omega|x^*, y) \quad \propto \quad f(x^*, x|y, \beta_1, \omega) f(\beta_1, \omega)$$

$$\propto \quad \left\{ \prod_{i=1}^{n} f(x_i^*|x_i) f(x_i|y_i, \beta_1, \omega) \right\} f(\beta_1, \omega)$$

$$\propto \quad \prod_{i=1}^{n} f(x_i^*|x_i) \times$$

$$\prod_{i=1}^{n} \frac{\exp\left[y_i \left\{\beta_0^*(\beta_1, \omega) + \beta_1 x_i\right\}\right]}{r + (1 - r) \exp\left\{\beta_0^*(\beta_1, \omega) + \beta_1 x_i\right\}} h(x_i|\omega) \times$$

$$f(\beta_1, \omega).$$

Upon reparameterizing from β_0^* to $\beta_0 = \beta_0^* + log(1 - r) - log(r)$, and ignoring multiplicative constants not depending on the unknowns (x, β_1, ω), this can be expressed as

$$f(x, \beta_1, \omega | x^*, y) \quad \propto \quad \prod_{i=1}^{n} f(x_i^* | x_i) \times$$

$$\prod_{i=1}^{n} \frac{\exp\left[y_i \left\{\beta_0(\beta_1, \omega) + \beta_1 x_i\right\}\right]}{1 + \exp\left\{\beta_0(\beta_1, \omega) + \beta_1 x_i\right\}} h(x_i|\omega) \times$$

$$f(\beta_1, \omega). \tag{4.37}$$

Here the constraint which determines β_0 as a function of (β_1, ω) is now expressed as

$$E_\omega \left\{\frac{1}{\beta_0 + \beta_1 X}\right\} = r,$$

which is readily solved numerically.

The important point is that (4.37) looks a lot like the posterior density which would arise in a prospective setting with $h(\cdot|\omega)$ as an exposure model, namely

$$f(x, \beta_0, \beta_1, \omega | x^*, y) \quad \propto \quad \prod_{i=1}^{n} f(x_i^* | x_i) \times$$

$$\prod_{i=1}^{n} \frac{\exp\left\{y_i(\beta_0 + \beta_1 x_i)\right\}}{1 + \exp(\beta_0 + \beta_1 x_i)} h(x_i|\omega) \times$$

$$f(\beta_0, \beta_1, \omega). \tag{4.38}$$

The difference is that β_0 is also an unknown parameter under (4.38), whereas it is a known function of the unknown parameters under (4.37). To see if this is a meaningful difference in practice we propose drawing a posterior sample of the parameters under (4.38) and then using *importance sampling* to make this sample represent the posterior (4.37). See Evans and Swartz (2000) for general discussion on the use of importance sampling for Bayesian inference. This approach is particularly attractive in the present scenario, as it is much easier to apply MCMC algorithms to (4.38) than to (4.37) given the constraint involved in the latter case.

A technical difficulty in applying importance sampling is that (4.38) is a distribution over $(x, \beta_0, \beta_1, \omega)$ whereas (4.37) is a distribution over (x, β_1, ω) only. To overcome this we artificially extend (4.37) to the larger space by appending the conditional distribution $\beta_0 | \beta_1, \omega, x \sim N(a_0 + a_1\beta_1, a_2^2)$ to (4.37) for some fixed (a_0, a_1, a_2). To minimize extra 'noise' in the importance weights we choose a as follows. We generate a preliminary sample from (4.38), and fit

scenario	post. mean	post. SD	rel. change
(i)	0.570 / 0.509	0.229 / 0.210	26.6%
(ii)	0.290 / 0.283	0.088 / 0.086	8.3%
(iii)	0.363 / 0.363	0.048 / 0.048	0.1%

Table 4.5 *Posterior means and standard deviations for β_1 in the example of Section 4.8. In each instance the first entry is based on the posterior arising from the prospective analysis, while the second entry corresponds to the retrospective analysis. Thus the first entry is computed from the MCMC sample while the second entry reflects the importance sampling adjustment. The reported relative change is the absolute difference between the two posterior means expressed as a percentage of the (prospective) posterior standard deviation. Scenarios (i), (ii), and (iii) involve increasing sample sizes, as described in the text.*

the postulated linear model for $\beta_0|\beta_1$ to the sampled values. Then (a_0, a_1) are taken to be the fitted coefficients and a_2 is taken to be the residual standard deviation. The idea here is to make the contrived distribution of $\beta_0|\beta_1$ under (4.37) as close as possible to the actual distribution of $\beta_0|\beta_1$ under (4.38). This limits the amount of extra noise introduced into the importance weights.

We try this procedure on a subset of the smoking and bladder cancer data from Section 4.4. As before, X^* and X are the self-reported and actual smoking exposures on the log pack-years scale, and we consider the measurement model $X^*|X \sim N(X, \tau^2)$ where $\tau = 0.5$. The pseudo-exposure model is simply taken to be normal with $\omega = (\alpha_0, \lambda^2)$ being the mean and variance. In the first instance we create dataset (i) by randomly selecting $n_0 = 100$ of the 5348 controls and $n_1 = 100$ of the 914 cases. Given these data, a posterior sample of size 500 is generated from (4.38) using MCMC as in Section 4.4. In fact this sample is obtained from every tenth of 5000 post burn-in MCMC iterations, in order to obtain a high-quality posterior sample with low serial correlation. Importance weights are determined by taking the ratio of the extended version of (4.37) to (4.38) for each sample point and then normalizing. The upper-left panel of Figure 4.8 plots the importance weights against the values of β_1. There does appear to be a substantial negative correlation between the weights and the values, implying that the posterior mean of β_1 under the retrospective analysis is smaller than under the prospective analysis. Indeed, Table 4.5 indicates the difference is substantial, as the two posterior means differ by about one-quarter of a posterior standard deviation. Thus the importance sampling is providing a nonnegligible adjustment to the prospective posterior distribution, to account for the fact that the data were collected retrospectively.

The same analysis is performed on dataset (ii) comprised of $n_0 = n_1 = 500$ randomly selected controls and cases, and on the full dataset (iii) of $n_0 = 5348$ controls and $n_1 = 914$ cases. Figure 4.8 and Table 4.5 indicate that the importance sampling adjustment becomes less pronounced as the sample sizes increase, to the point of being negligible for the full dataset. This is in keeping

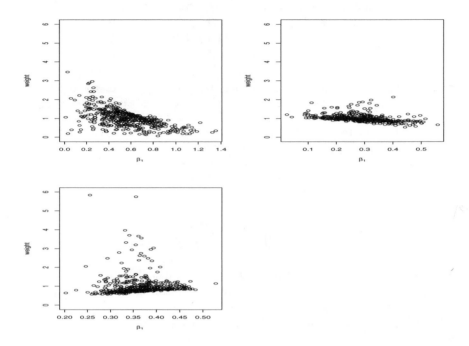

Figure 4.8 *Importance weights in the example of Section 4.8. In each scenario the importance weights for the posterior sample of 500 realizations are plotted against the sample values of β_1. The weights are normalized to sum to 500, so that one is the mean weight. Scenarios (i), (ii), and (iii) involve increasing sample sizes, as described in the text.*

with the aforementioned large-sample justifications for analyzing retrospective data as if it were collected prospectively.

4.9 Comparison with Non-Bayesian Approaches

There is a vast literature on methods to adjust for mismeasurement of continuous explanatory variables, and it is beyond the scope of this book to provide a comprehensive review of this work. Nevertheless, it seems prudent to remark on the relationship between Bayes-MCMC methods as described in this chapter and other methods.

For inference in measurement error scenarios, the nearest cousin to Bayesian estimation is maximum likelihood estimation. Both approaches require a likelihood function arising from fully specified measurement, outcome, and exposure models. In particular, the likelihood function is obtained by integrating over the true but unobserved explanatory variable. As alluded to in Section 4.2, often this integration cannot be done explicitly in closed-form. In such cases, one possibility is to evaluate the likelihood function using a numerical integration scheme, so that iterative schemes to maximize the likelihood function can be employed. For instance, Crouch and Spiegelman (1990) suggest a particular numerical integration scheme to handle a logistic regression outcome model with normal measurement and exposure models.

As we have seen, for Bayesian inference MCMC techniques provide a general approach to doing the requisite integration 'behind the scenes.' For a likelihood analysis the *expectation-maximization* (EM) algorithm can play a similar role, with an E-step that updates an expected log-likelihood by averaging over the unobserved explanatory variable given the observed quantities and the current parameter values, and a M-step that updates parameter values by maximizing the expected log-likelihood. In general, by iterating back and forth between E and M steps the algorithm converges to parameter values corresponding to at least a local maxima of the likelihood function.

One issue in applying the EM algorithm to measurement error problems is that the expectations to be computed in the E-step may themselves not have closed-form expressions, so that approximations must be used. Schafer (1987) discusses approximations specific to a measurement error model, while more generally there is a considerable literature on Monte Carlo approximations to the E-step. Also, it requires extra effort to obtain standard errors when maximum likelihood estimates are obtained via the EM algorithm (Louis 1982). These limitations likely contribute to the dearth of literature on likelihood-based inference in measurement error problems noted by Carroll, Ruppert and Stefanski (1995). Since Bayes-MCMC inference does not require approximations (or more precisely it can be made as exact as desired by increasing the Monte Carlo sample size), and since uncertainty assessments are obtained without any extra effort, one can argue that the Bayes-MCMC approach is the easiest route to likelihood-based inference in measurement error models.

There are a number of inferential approaches to measurement error problems that are designed to avoid the full specification of measurement, outcome, and exposure models. In particular, much of the literature addresses methods that avoid the explicit construction of an exposure model. Sometimes such approaches are referred to as *functional* methods, whereas *structural* methods do make assumptions about the exposure distribution. Two quite general and popular functional approaches involve *regression calibration* and *simulation extrapolation*, both of which we describe briefly.

While special cases of regression calibration appear earlier (notably Rosner, Willett and Spiegelman 1989 for a logistic regression outcome model), the general idea is discussed by Carroll and Stefanski (1990) and Gleser (1990). Consider outcome variable Y, actual exposure X, mismeasured exposure X^*, and other precisely measured explanatory variables Z. The central idea of regression calibration is quite straightforward. Naively using (X^*, Z) instead of the desired but unobservable (X, Z) as explanatory variables in fitting the outcome model leads to biased inference in general. However, at least approximately unbiased inference can arise if the explanatory variables are taken to be $\{\hat{m}(X^*, Z), Z\}$, where $\hat{m}(X^*, Z)$ is an estimate of $m(X^*, Z) = E(X|X^*, Z)$. That is, a 'best-guess' X value is imputed for each subject, given the values of X^* and Z. Moreover, in some scenarios $m(\cdot)$ can be estimated without the specification of an exposure model. In particular, with a validation subsample one can directly regress X^* on (X, Z) and use the fitted relationship as $\hat{m}(\cdot)$, which is then applied to impute best-guess X values for the main sample subjects. It is interesting to note, however, that there is no obvious analogue of regression calibration in the ostensibly simpler scenario of a known measurement model but no validation subsample.

It is straightforward to see how regression calibration works in the simple setting of a linear outcome model. Say $E(Y|X, Z) = \beta_0 + \beta_1 X + \beta_2 Z$, and X^* is conditionally independent of (Y, Z) given X. Then

$$
\begin{aligned}
E(Y|X^*, Z) &= E\{E(Y|X^*, X, Z)|X^*, Z)\} \\
&= E\{\beta_0 + \beta_1 X + \beta_2 Z|X^*, Z) \\
&= \beta_0 + \beta_1 E(X|X^*, Z) + \beta_2 Z,
\end{aligned}
$$

so that in principle one can estimate $(\beta_0, \beta_1, \beta_2)$ by regression of Y on $m(X^*, Z)$ and Z. Rosner, Willett and Spiegelman (1989) and Rosner, Spiegelman and Willett (1990) demonstrate that the same general approach works reasonably with logistic regression models for binary outcomes, provided the measurement error is relatively modest in magnitude.

A clear difference between regression calibration and Bayes-MCMC inference is that the former is a two-stage procedure: first guessed values for X are imputed using only (X^*, Z), then the imputed values are used as regressors in the outcome model for Y. In contrast, the Bayes analysis involves simultaneous consideration of (X^*, Y, X, Z). In general the two-stage procedure will be somewhat inefficient relative to a Bayes or likelihood procedure, though this does not seem to have been looked at closely in the literature. On the other hand, of course, the lack of need for an exposure model does make the regression calibration approach less susceptible to bias arising from model misspecification.

Another issue with the two-stage nature of regression-calibration involves the propagation of uncertainty. The usual standard errors obtained when fitting the outcome model will be too small, as they will neglect the uncertainty arising because the imputed X values are not the true X values. There is some scope for correcting this via appropriate mathematical expansions, or more generally via bootstrapping (Carroll, Ruppert and Stefanski 1995). In contrast, a nice feature of Bayes-MCMC analysis is that appropriate uncertainty assessments are built-in to the analysis, with no special effort required to extract them. In particular, Bayes-MCMC inference averages over plausible values of X in light of the data, rather than imputing a single best-guess and then proceeding as if this guess is correct.

Another quite general approach to measurement error correction is simulation extrapolation (SIMEX), as first suggested by Cook and Stefanski (1995), and discussed at length by Carroll, Ruppert and Stefanski (1995). The basic idea is very simple and intuitively appealing. Say that for the actual dataset at hand the measurement error variance $Var(X^*|X)$ is estimated or known to be τ_0^2, and let $\hat{\theta}(\tau_0^2)$ be the naive (i.e., unadjusted for measurement error) estimate of the parameter of interest θ. It is simple to add further measurement error to an already noisy predictor, so one can create a new dataset in which the measurement error variance is $\tau_1^2 > \tau_0^2$ simply by adding $N(0, \tau_1^2 - \tau_0^2)$ noise to the original X^* values. Thus the naive estimate in the new dataset is $\hat{\theta}(\tau_1^2)$. One can continue to add further noise and thereby determine $\hat{\theta}(\tau^2)$ at numerous values of $\tau^2 > \tau_0^2$. In particular, one could consider fitting a smooth line or curve to these points in order to represent $\hat{\theta}(\tau^2)$ as a function of τ^2. By extrapolating this curve to values of τ *smaller* than τ_0^2, one considers estimates of θ under hypothetical reductions in measurement error. In particular, the extrapolated value of $\hat{\theta}(0)$ is taken as an estimate of θ which is fully corrected for measurement error.

Thus SIMEX provides a route to measurement error adjustment which is very easy to understand and implement. In addition, it does not require the specification of an exposure model. On the other hand, it does require the choice of a functional form for $\hat{\theta}$ as a function of τ^2 in the requisite curve-fitting procedure. There is always a danger in extrapolating a function beyond the range where function values are observed, so that the extrapolated value of $\hat{\theta}(0)$ can be sensitive to the choice of functional form. Kuchenhoff and Carroll (1997) provide an example of this, in a relatively complex setting involving segmented regression. Thus the tradeoff is that SIMEX avoids the potential pitfall of bias due to a poorly specified exposure model, but introduces the potential pitfall of bias due to a poor extrapolation. Neither problem is readily diagnosed from the observed data, so it is hard to make a definitive comparison between SIMEX and likelihood-based inference. Of course with correctly specified models likelihood-based inference will necessarily be more efficient than SIMEX estimation. In the specialized context of Kuchenhoff and Carroll (1997), maximum likelihood estimators are found to have considerably smaller variance than both SIMEX and regression calibration estimators.

While regression calibration and SIMEX are relatively general functional methods for measurement error, there are numerous other approaches which are typically aimed at quite specific modelling scenarios. Carroll, Ruppert and Stefanski (1995) discuss a number of such methods. Historically structural approaches involving an exposure model have not been as popular, though they have received increased attention recently, perhaps in large part due to the advent of MCMC techniques. While the potential for exposure model misspecification is an issue, arguably it has been exaggerated as a rationale for using functional approaches. In addition to the transparent straightforwardness of working with fully specified (i.e., structural) probability models, there is always the possibility of using more flexible exposure models, as discussed earlier in the chapter. It also seems strange that exposure model misspecification receives so much attention when both structural and functional approaches are prone to misspecification of the measurement and outcome models. We return to this point at greater length in Section 6.2.

4.10 Summary

We hope this chapter illustrates that the Bayes-MCMC machinery provides a general and powerful way to adjust inferences to account for measurement error in explanatory variables. In particular, the recipe is quite clear: make the best specifications of measurement, outcome, and exposure models one can, along with appropriate prior distributions for the unknown parameters in these models. Then apply MCMC to sample from the posterior distribution of unknown parameters and unobserved variables given the observed variables. Inferential summaries obtained from such a posterior sample will be adjusted in a principled way to account for the measurement error.

As with most statistical techniques, of course, the devil can be in the details. On the technical side, it is not always easy to choose or devise a particular MCMC algorithm that works well on the problem at hand. On the modelling side, sometimes the need for three fully specified models and priors may seem arduous, particularly in relation to some non-Bayesian techniques which seem to entail fewer assumptions. On balance the author contends that the advantages of the Bayes-MCMC approach more than outweigh the disadvantages, though admittedly there is scope for further research on the comparative utility of various methods.

4.11 Mathematical Details

4.11.1 Full Conditional Distributions in the Example of Section 4.2

Consider the first study design in the example of Section 4.2. With the assumed model and prior distributions, the posterior distribution (4.7) for the unobserved quantities $U = (x_R, \beta, \alpha, \tau^2, \sigma^2, \lambda^2)$ given the observed quantities $O = (x^*, x_C, y, z)$ becomes

$$
\begin{aligned}
f(U|O) \quad \propto \quad & \left(\frac{1}{\tau^2}\right)^{n/2} \exp\left(-\frac{\sum_{i=1}^{n}(x_i^* - x_i)^2}{2\tau^2}\right) \times \\
& \left(\frac{1}{\sigma^2}\right)^{n/2} \exp\left(-\frac{\sum_{i=1}^{n}(y_i - \beta_0 - \beta_1 x_i - \beta_2 z_i)^2}{2\sigma^2}\right) \times \\
& \left(\frac{1}{\lambda^2}\right)^{n/2} \exp\left(-\frac{\sum_{i=1}^{n}(x_i - \alpha_0 - \alpha_1 z_i)^2}{2\lambda^2}\right) \times \\
& \left(\frac{1}{\tau^2}\right)^{(0.5+1)} \exp\left(-\frac{(0.5)}{\tau^2}\right) \times \\
& \left(\frac{1}{\sigma^2}\right)^{(0.5+1)} \exp\left(-\frac{(0.5)}{\sigma^2}\right) \times \\
& \left(\frac{1}{\lambda^2}\right)^{(0.5+1)} \exp\left(-\frac{(0.5)}{\lambda^2}\right).
\end{aligned}
$$

By viewing this expression as a function of one individual unobserved quantity at a time we can easily 'read off' the full conditional distributions. We use a complement notation, so that generically ν^C would denote all the unobserved quantities other than ν along with all the observed quantities. For instance,

$$\alpha | \alpha^C \quad \sim \quad N_2 \left\{ (A'A)^{-1} A'x, \lambda^2 (A'A)^{-1} \right\},$$

where A is the $n \times 2$ design matrix with i-th row $(1, z_i)$. Similarly,

$$\beta | \beta^C \quad \sim \quad N \left\{ (B'B)^{-1} B'y, \sigma^2 (B'B)^{-1} \right\},$$

where B is the $n \times 3$ design matrix with i-th row $(1, x_i, z_i)$. Note in particular that B depends on x_R. For the variance components we have,

$$\lambda^2 | \lambda^{2 \, C} \quad \sim \quad IG \left\{ (n+1)/2, (\|x - A\alpha\|^2 + 1)/2 \right\},$$

$$\sigma^2 | \sigma^{2 \, C} \quad \sim \quad IG \left\{ (n+1)/2, (\|y - A\beta\|^2 + 1)/2 \right\},$$

and

$$\tau^2 | \tau^{2 \, C} \quad \sim \quad IG \left\{ (n+1)/2, (\|x^* - x\|^2 + 1)/2 \right\}.$$

Finally, we also need full conditional distributions for the components of x_R. If i indexes a reduced case then viewing the posterior density as a function of x_i alone gives the conditional distribution of $x_i | x_i^C$ as normal, with

$$E \left(x_i | x_i^C \right) \quad = \quad \frac{(1/\tau^2) x_i^* + (\beta_1^2/\sigma^2) \{ (y - \beta_0 - \beta_2 z_i)/\beta_1 \}}{(1/\tau^2) + (\beta_1^2/\sigma^2)}$$

and

$$Var \left(x_i | x_i^C \right) \quad = \quad \frac{1}{(1/\tau^2) + (\beta_1^2/\sigma^2)}.$$

Thus to implement the Gibbs sampler in this example we simply need to sample repeatedly from these full conditional distributions. Thus standard routines to generate realizations from normal and inverse gamma distributions are all that is required.

In the case of the second study design, the full conditionals for α, β, σ^2, and λ^2 are exactly as above. But now

$$\tau^2 | \tau^{2 \, C} \quad \sim \quad IG \left\{ 0.5 + n, 0.5 + \|x_1^* - x\|^2 + \|x_2^* - x\|^2 \right\},$$

and for reduced cases $x_i | x_i^C$ is normal with

$$E \left(x_i | x_i^C \right) \quad = \quad \frac{(2/\tau^2) \bar{x}_i^* + (\beta_1^2/\sigma^2) \{ (y - \beta_0 - \beta_2' z_i)/\beta_1 \}}{(2/\tau^2) + (\beta_1^2/\sigma^2)},$$

and

$$Var \left(x_i | x_i^C \right) \quad = \quad \frac{1}{(2/\tau^2) + (\beta_1^2/\sigma^2)},$$

where $\bar{x}_i^* = (x_{1i}^* + x_{2i}^*)/2$ is simply the average of the two X^* measurements for the i-th subject.

4.11.2 MCMC for the Models of Sections 4.4 and 4.5

In applying MCMC to logistic regression models we must typically update a vector of coefficients β having a full conditional density of the form

$$f(\beta|\beta^C) \quad \propto \quad \prod_{i=1}^{n} \frac{\exp\{y_i(\beta_0 + \beta_1 x_i + \beta_2' z_i)\}}{1 + \exp\{\beta_0 + \beta_1 x_i + \beta_2' z_i\}} f(\beta), \qquad (4.39)$$

where we have followed the notation of (4.23). We elucidate both a good but expensive update and a poor but cheap update. If we are willing to use an iterative numerical routine to maximize the logistic regression log-likelihood, then we can sample a candidate β vector from the normal distribution with mean and variance chosen to match the log-likelihood's mode and curvature at the mode. Note that by doing so we are generating a candidate value that does not depend on the current value, which might be referred to as an *independence MH algorithm*. Standard asymptotic theory dictates that this normal distribution will typically be an excellent approximation to (4.39), as long as the sample size is moderately large. In turn this implies a very high Metropolis-Hastings acceptance rate for the update. The combination of a high acceptance rate and a candidate-generating distribution which does not depend on the current value of β makes for a very efficient MCMC algorithm. However, maximizing the likelihood will take considerable CPU time, and since x is updated in between the updates to β, it is necessary to re-maximize every time β is to be updated. Thus this is a good but slow update.

A much cheaper update not involving maximization is the random-walk MH algorithm applied to one component of β at a time. While such an update is fast, it has several drawbacks. First, it is necessary to set a tuning parameter (the jump size) for each component of β. Second, this algorithm may mix quite slowly. There is some scope for improving the mixing by centering the explanatory variables (i.e., forcing them to have mean zero), as discussed by Gilks and Roberts (1996) and Roberts and Sahu (1997), although we have not found this to be a panacea. As well, centering is slightly less straightforward in the present scenario where x changes from update to update of β.

In implementing updates to logistic regression parameters we tend to compromise and use both slow and fast updates. In particular, we preserve the desired stationary distribution by randomly choosing the update method immediately prior to each update. That is, with some small probability a slow update is performed, but otherwise a fast update is carried out. Empirically this seems to be a decent overall strategy which achieves both reasonable mixing and reasonable execution time.

4.11.3 Proof of Result 4.1

Upon expressing β_1 in terms of the collapsed model parameterization we have

$$l_1 \quad = \quad lsl(\tilde{\beta}_1) \left(1 + \frac{\tau^2}{lsl(\tilde{\lambda}^2) - \tau^2}\right), \qquad (4.40)$$

where $lsl(\tilde{\beta}_1)$ and $lsl(\tilde{\lambda}^2)$ are the large-sample limits of Bayes or maximum likelihood estimators of $\tilde{\beta}_1$ and $\tilde{\lambda}^2$ respectively. Since $lsl(\tilde{\beta}_1)$ will be the large-sample limit of the X^* coefficient in regressing Y on $(1, X^*, Z)$, Result 2.1 gives immediately

$$lsl(\tilde{\beta}_1) \;=\; \frac{l_0}{1 + \tau^2 / \{Var(X)(1 - Cor(X, Z)^2)\}}. \tag{4.41}$$

On the other hand, standard large-sample theory gives the limit of the estimated residual variance for $X^*|Z$ under possible model misspecification as

$$
\begin{aligned}
lsl(\tilde{\lambda}^2) \;&=\; Var(X^*)\left\{1 - Cor(X^*, Z)^2\right\} \\
&=\; Var(X)\left\{1 - Cor(X, Z)^2\right\} + \tau^2,
\end{aligned} \tag{4.42}
$$

where the second equality follows from conditional independence of X^* and (Y, Z) given X, along with $E(X^*|X) = X$ and $Var(X^*|X) = \tau^2$. Plugging (4.41) and (4.42) into (4.40) gives $l_1 = l_0$, as desired.

4.11.4 Proof of Result 4.2

Here we use an alternate notation for the parameters in the collapsed model, for the sake of more compact mathematical expressions. In particular, the collapsed model corresponding to this full model can be parameterized by $\theta = (\gamma_0, \gamma_1, \nu, \phi_0, \omega)$, with $Y|X^* \sim N(\gamma_0 + \gamma_1 X^*, \nu)$ and $X^* \sim N(\phi_0, \omega)$. Moreover, β_1 in the full model can be estimated as $\hat{\beta}_1 = g\left(\hat{\theta}\right)$, where

$$g(\theta) \;=\; \gamma_1 \left(1 + \frac{\tau^2}{\omega - \tau^2}\right).$$

Straightforward calculation gives the score vector for the collapsed model as

$$s(\theta; X^*, Y) \;=\; \begin{pmatrix} \nu^{-1}(Y - \gamma_0 - \gamma_1 X^*) \\ \nu^{-1}(Y - \gamma_0 - \gamma_1 X^*)X^* \\ -(0.5)\nu^{-1} + (0.5)\nu^{-2}(Y - \gamma_0 - \gamma_1 X^*)^2 \\ \omega^{-1}(X^* - \phi_0) \\ -(0.5)\omega^{-1} + (0.5)\omega^{-2}(X^* - \phi_0)^2 \end{pmatrix}. \tag{4.43}$$

For the time being assume that X has been scaled so that $E(X) = 0$ and $Var(X) = 1$. The value $\theta = \theta^*$ solving $E\{s(\theta; X^*, Y)\} = 0$ is given by

$$
\begin{aligned}
\gamma_0 \;&=\; \beta_0 \\
\gamma_1 \;&=\; \beta_1/(1 + \tau^2) \\
\nu \;&=\; \sigma^2 + \beta_1^2 \tau^2/(1 + \tau^2) \\
\phi_0 \;&=\; 0 \\
\omega \;&=\; 1 + \tau^2,
\end{aligned}
$$

which does not depend on the actual distribution of X (above and beyond the fixed first and second moments). Standard large-sample theory for misspecified models (e.g., White 1982) implies that Bayesian and maximum likelihood estimators of θ converge to θ^*. Moreover, the asymptotic variance of such an estimator is given as $A^{-1}BA^{-1}$, where

$$A = -E\{s'(\theta^*; X^*, Y)\}$$

and

$$B = E\left[\{s(\theta^*; X^*, Y)\}\{s(\theta^*; X^*, Y)\}'\right].$$

Under the assumed scaling of X it is simple to compute

$$A = \begin{pmatrix} \nu^{-1} & 0 & 0 & 0 & 0 \\ & \nu^{-1}(1+\tau^2) & 0 & 0 & 0 \\ & & (0.5)\nu^{-2} & 0 & 0 \\ & & & (1+\tau^2)^{-1} & 0 \\ & & & & 0.5(1+\tau^2)^{-2} \end{pmatrix}.$$

Since A is diagonal and $g(\theta)$ depends only on (γ_1, ω), the only elements of B that must be computed are B_{22}, B_{55}, and B_{25}. Towards this end, note that we can write

$$Y - \gamma_0 - \gamma_1 X^* = \beta_1\left(\frac{\tau^2}{1+\tau^2}\right)X + \epsilon_1$$

and

$$X^* = X + \epsilon_2,$$

where

$$\begin{pmatrix} \epsilon_1 \\ \epsilon_2 \end{pmatrix} \sim N\left(\begin{bmatrix} 0 \\ 0 \end{bmatrix}, \begin{bmatrix} \sigma^2 + \gamma_1^2\tau^2 & -\gamma_1\tau^2 \\ -\gamma_1\tau^2 & \tau^2 \end{bmatrix}\right)$$

independently of X. Starting from (4.43) this leads to

$$B_{22} = A_{22} + \frac{(\beta_1 - \gamma_1)^2}{\nu^2}\delta$$

$$B_{55} = A_{55} + \frac{1}{4(1+\tau^2)^4}\delta$$

$$B_{25} = A_{25} + \frac{\beta_1 - \gamma_1}{2\nu\omega^2}\delta,$$

where

$$\delta = E\left(X^4\right) - 3.$$

Bearing in mind the standardization, if X has a normal distribution then $\delta = 0$. Of course theory dictates that $B = A$ in this case of a correctly specified model, as witnessed by the above equations.

Now from the Delta method we have the asymptotic variance of $\hat{\beta}_1 = g(\hat{\theta})$ as

$$\begin{aligned} Avar\left[g(\theta)\right] = \ & (1+\tau^2)^2 (A^{-1}BA^{-1})_{22} + \\ & \gamma_1^2\tau^4(A^{-1}BA^{-1})_{55} + \\ & -2\gamma_1(1+\tau^2)\tau^2(A^{-1}BA^{-1})_{25}. \end{aligned}$$

This specializes to

$$
\begin{aligned}
Avar\,[g(\theta)] \;=\;& (1+\tau^2)^2 \left\{ \frac{\sigma^2}{1+\tau^2} + \frac{\beta_1^2 \tau^2}{(1+\tau^2)^2} + \frac{\beta_1^2 \tau^4}{(1+\tau^2)^4}\delta \right\} + \\
& \frac{\beta_1^2 \tau^4}{(1+\tau^2)^2} \left\{ 2(1+\tau^2)^2 + \delta \right\} + \\
& (-2)\beta_1 \tau^2 \left\{ \frac{\beta_1 \tau^2}{(1+\tau^2)^2}\delta \right\}.
\end{aligned}
$$

Clearly the terms involving δ cancel, so that the asymptotic variance of the estimator does not depend on the actual distribution of the standardized X. In particular,

$$
Avar\,[g(\theta)] \;=\; (1+\tau^2)\sigma^2 + \beta_1^2 \tau^2 + 2\beta_1^2 \tau^4. \tag{4.44}
$$

Finally, it remains to generalize this expression to the case where X is not standardized. From invariance considerations it is straightforward to determine that the more general expression can be determined from (4.44) by first substituting $\beta_1 Var(X)$ for β_1 and $\tau^2/Var(X)$ for τ^2, and then dividing the entire expression by $Var(X)$. This results in (4.30), as desired.

It is interesting to note that misspecification does affect the asymptotic variance of estimators of γ_1 and ω, as these variances do depend on δ. However misspecification also induces dependence between the two estimators, so that when they are combined to estimate β_1 there is a seemingly remarkable cancellation of the terms involving δ.

CHAPTER 5

Adjusting for Mismeasured Categorical Variables

The previous chapter described how to carry out analyses which adjust for mismeasurement in continuous explanatory variables, to avoid the sorts of biases described in Chapter 2. Now we turn attention to analyses which adjust for mismeasurement in binary explanatory variables, to avoid the sorts of biases described in Chapter 3. In Sections 5.1 and 5.2 we consider a binary outcome and a binary explanatory variable, with data arising from a case-control study design. In the first instance the extent of misclassification is known exactly, whereas Section 5.2 extends to the more practical case of imperfect prior information about the misclassification. Section 5.3 moves on to consider situations where there is little or no prior information about the misclassification, but several different noisy measurements of the explanatory variable are available. Section 5.4 extends further to situations where additional precisely measured explanatory variables are measured. Some brief concluding remarks appear in Section 5.5, while mathematical details are gathered in Section 5.6.

5.1 A Simple Scenario

Say that the relationship between a binary outcome variable Y and a binary exposure variable V is of interest, but a surrogate binary variable V^* is measured in lieu of V. As a simple initial scenario, say that data are collected via a retrospective case-control study, with n_0 subjects sampled at random from the control $(Y = 0)$ population, and n_1 subjects sampled at random from the case $(Y = 1)$ population. Thus samples from the conditional distribution of $V^*|Y$ are obtained, for both $Y = 0$ and $Y = 1$. Of course a naive analysis which treats V^* as if it were V will typically yield biased inferences concerning the relationship between V and Y, as described in Chapter 3. However, if enough is known about the mismeasurement process then it can be quite straightforward to make inferences which account for the mismeasurement. Particularly, say that the distribution of $V^*|V, Y$ is known completely. Then, paralleling the analyses presented in Chapter 4, inference could proceed by including each subject's unobserved V variable as an unknown quantity described by the posterior distribution. In fact, an even simpler approach to Bayesian analysis suffices in the present scenario. It is easy to directly simulate draws from the posterior distribution of the unknown parameters given the observed data, without incorporating the V variables explicitly.

To be more specific, let r_0 and r_1 be the prevalence of exposure in the control and case populations respectively. That is, the chance that a sampled control subject is exposed is $r_0 = Pr(V = 1|Y = 0)$ and the chance that a sampled case subject is exposed is $r_1 = Pr(V = 1|Y = 1)$. As alluded to in Chapter 3, usually the parameter of interest for describing the association between V and Y is the odds-ratio

$$\Psi = \frac{r_1/(1 - r_1)}{r_0/(1 - r_0)}. \tag{5.1}$$

Of course it is well known that Ψ has a dual interpretation as both the ratio of odds that $Y = 1$ given $V = 1$ to odds that $Y = 1$ given $V = 0$, and the ratio of odds that $V = 1$ given $Y = 1$ to odds that $V = 1$ given $Y = 0$. It is often convenient to think in terms of the log odds-ratio which, for future reference, we denote as $\psi = \log \Psi$.

Under the common assumption of nondifferential misclassification, whereby the conditional distribution of $V^*|V, Y$ does not actually depend on Y, the magnitude of misclassification is characterized in terms of sensitivity and specificity. Whereas in Chapter 3 we used (SN, SP) to denote these quantities, now we use (p, q) for the sake of compactness in mathematical expressions. That is, $p = Pr(V^* = 1|V = 1)$ is the sensitivity and $q = Pr(V^* = 0|V = 0)$ is the specificity. In the present scenario we take (p, q) to be known. Of course in many real scenarios the assumptions of nondifferential misclassification and known sensitivity and specificity will be questionable at best. As noted in Chapter 3, the nondifferential assumption can be particularly tenuous in a retrospective study, particularly when the surrogate V^* is based on subject self-report. Moreover, while investigators may have reasonable estimates or guesses for the values of p and q, scenarios where these values are actually known are rare. Indeed, even if it is reasonable to think p and q are 'known' from a previous study in which both V^* and V were measured, there may be questions about whether (p, q) are transportable across different study populations. Thus one must be circumspect about the extent to which the illustrative analysis in this section is realistic.

In the simple situation at hand, adjusting estimated odds-ratios to account for misclassification has been discussed at length in the literature (see, for instance, Barron 1977, Greenland and Kleinbaum 1983, Morrissey and Spiegelman 1999). Here we present a Bayesian approach to such adjustment. Whereas most of the discussion in the epidemiology literature involves only the adjustment of point estimates, the Bayesian approach has the advantage of automatically adjusting interval estimates simultaneously.

The observed data can be summarized by (S_0, S_1), where S_0 is the number of the n_0 cases who are *apparently* exposed in the sense that $V^* = 1$, while similarly S_1 is the number of the n_1 cases who are apparently exposed. Since an apparent exposure can result from the correct classification of an exposed subject or from the incorrect classification of an unexposed subject, it immediately follows that $S_i \sim Binomial(n_i, \theta_i)$, where

$$\theta_i = Pr(V^* = 1|Y = i)$$

$$\begin{aligned} &= Pr(V = 1|Y = i)Pr(V^* = 1|V = 1, Y = i) \; + \\ &\quad Pr(V = 0|Y = i)Pr(V^* = 1|V = 0, Y = i) \\ &= r_i p + (1 - r_i)(1 - q) \end{aligned} \qquad (5.2)$$

is the probability of *apparent* exposure given $Y = i$. Via (5.2) one can regard either (r_0, r_1) or (θ_0, θ_1) as the unknown parameters in the statistical model for the observed data. In going back and forth between these two parameterizations, note that while each r_i can take on any value between zero and one, each θ_i is necessarily constrained to lie in the interval from $l(p, q) = \min\{p, 1 - q\}$ to $r(p, q) = \max\{p, 1 - q\}$. Note as well that in the second parameterization the odds-ratio is expressed as

$$\Psi = \frac{(\theta_1 + q - 1)/(p - \theta_1)}{(\theta_0 + q - 1)/(p - \theta_0)}. \qquad (5.3)$$

In the absence of well-formed prior information an investigator might reasonably take the priors for r_0 and r_1 to be uniform distributions on the unit interval, with an assumption of prior independence. That is, $r_i \sim U(0, 1)$ independently for $i = 0, 1$. Clearly this implies that $\theta_i \sim U\{l(p, q), r(p, q)\}$ independently for $i = 0, 1$. Whereas a uniform prior on the unit interval and a binomial likelihood lead to a Beta posterior, a uniform prior on a sub-interval of $(0, 1)$ will yield a Beta distribution truncated to the sub-interval as the posterior distribution. Particularly, θ_0 and θ_1 are conditionally independent given the data (S_0, S_1), with $\theta_i|S_0, S_1$ following the $Beta(S_i + 1, n_i - S_i + 1)$ distribution truncated to $\{l(p, q), r(p, q)\}$. Thus it is trivial to simulate from the posterior distribution in the θ parameterization, and thereby obtain a Monte Carlo posterior sample for Ψ via (5.3). We emphasize that this is direct rather than MCMC simulation, so there are no concerns about convergence or mixing associated with the posterior sample.

To test this inferential scheme four synthetic datasets are simulated, each with sample sizes $n_0 = n_1 = 2500$. Datasets (i) and (ii) are based on the same retrospective samples of $V|Y$, with exposure prevalences $(r_0, r_1) = (0.2, 0.25)$. The surrogate V^* values arise from $(p, q) = (0.95, 0.9)$ in (i), and from $(p, q) = (0.85, 0.9)$ in (ii). Datasets (iii) and (iv) are generated with lower underlying prevalences of $(r_0, r_1) = (0.05, 0.0656)$, to mimic the common use of case-control analysis when faced with relatively rare exposures. The misclassification arises from $(p, q) = (0.95, 0.90)$ in (iii) and $(p, q) = (0.85, 0.90)$ in (iv), thereby matching the first two datasets. Note that both choices of prevalences (r_0, r_1) give an odds-ratio of $\Psi = 1.333$, and consequently a log odds-ratio of $\psi = 0.288$. Both the actual exposure totals and the apparent exposure totals for the four datasets appear in Table 5.1

Figure 5.1 displays the posterior distribution of the log odds-ratio ψ for each dataset, as determined in the manner described above. We refer to this as the *adjusted* posterior distribution in the sense that the analysis is adjusted to account for the misclassification. For the sake of comparison, both the *naive* and *ideal* posterior distributions of the log odds-ratio are also presented. The naive posterior results from ignoring the misclassification and treating the

	number actually exposed		number apparently exposed	
dataset	control	case	control	case
(i)	512/2500	641/2500	660/2500	773/2500
(ii)	512/2500	641/2500	637/2500	732/2500
(iii)	133/2500	175/2500	336/2500	394/2500
(iv)	133/2500	175/2500	321/2500	377/2500

Table 5.1 *Summary of the synthetic datasets considered in Section 5.1 Both the number of actual exposures and the number of apparent exposures are given for each sample. The underlying prevalences (r_0, r_1) and classification probabilities (p, q) are given in the text.*

surrogate exposure status V^* as if it were the actual exposure status V. In terms of the analysis described above, the naive posterior distribution arises from incorrectly assuming that $p = q = 1$. Alternately, the ideal posterior distribution results when V itself can be observed and used as the exposure variable, in which case V^* can be discarded. Of course we only have the luxury of determining the ideal posterior distribution because we simulate the data and thus have measurements of V. Thus the ideal posterior is of interest only for the sake of comparison and assessment of how much inferences are weakened because of misclassification.

For all four datasets the mode of the naive posterior distribution lies closer to zero than that of the ideal posterior distribution. Thus the attenuation that results from ignoring the misclassification is evident. In datasets (i) and (ii) the modes of both the adjusted and ideal posterior distributions are close to the true value of ψ, but the adjusted distribution is slightly wider than the ideal distribution. This reflects the loss of information associated with misclassification. In datasets (iii) and (iv) the adjusted posterior distribution is both wider and shifted to the right in relation to the ideal posterior distribution, with the discrepancy between the adjusted and ideal posteriors being comparable in magnitude to the discrepancy between the naive and ideal posteriors. Thus for datasets (i) and (ii) the adjusted analysis is clearly better than the naive analysis, while the benefit of adjustment is less obvious for datasets (iii) and (iv).

To investigate the benefit associated with adjustment more thoroughly, we turn to some simple comparisons based on asymptotic estimator performance. Let $\hat{\psi}_I$, $\hat{\psi}_A$, and $\hat{\psi}_N$ be estimators of ψ based on the ideal, adjusted, and naive posterior distributions respectively. For the sake of argument say these estimators are modes of the respective posterior distributions, but it is well known that posterior means or medians have the same asymptotic performance, and in particular all these estimators are asymptotically equivalent to the maximum likelihood estimator.

In the case of the ideal analysis, one has a correctly specified model and

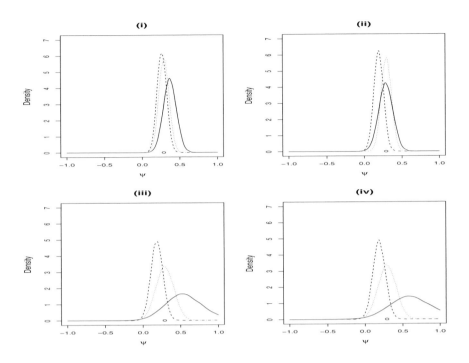

Figure 5.1 *Naive, corrected, and ideal posterior distributions of the log odds-ratio based on the four synthetic datasets given in Table 5.1. For each dataset the dashed curve corresponds to the naive analysis, the solid curve to the adjusted analysis, and the dotted curve to the ideal analysis.*

hence no bias asymptotically. Considering sample proportions of actual exposure we have $Var(\hat{r}_i) = n_i^{-1} r_i (1 - r_i)$. Applying the 'delta method' to the logarithm of (5.1) then gives

$$
\begin{aligned}
MSE(\hat{\psi}_I) &\approx Var(\hat{\psi}_I) \\
&\approx \frac{1}{n_0 r_0 (1 - r_0)} + \frac{1}{n_1 r_1 (1 - r_1)}.
\end{aligned}
\tag{5.4}
$$

Similarly, the adjusted analysis involves no bias asymptotically, provided correct values of p and q are specified. Considering sample proportions of apparent exposure we have $Var(\hat{\theta}_i) = n_i^{-1} \theta_i (1 - \theta_i)$. Viewing $\hat{\psi}_A$ as a function of $(\hat{\theta}_0, \hat{\theta}_1)$ according to (5.3) and then applying the delta method gives

$$
\begin{aligned}
MSE(\hat{\psi}_A) &\approx Var(\hat{\psi}_A) \\
&\approx \left\{ \frac{p + q - 1}{(\theta_0 + q - 1)(p - \theta_0)} \right\}^2 \frac{\theta_0 (1 - \theta_0)}{n_0} + \\
&\quad \left\{ \frac{p + q - 1}{(\theta_1 + q - 1)(p - \theta_1)} \right\}^2 \frac{\theta_1 (1 - \theta_1)}{n_1}.
\end{aligned}
\tag{5.5}
$$

Of course this expression could be re-cast in terms of (r_0, r_1) rather than (θ_0, θ_1), although doing so does not yield any obvious insights in terms of comparison with (5.4).

Finally, the naive analysis does involve a bias, with estimates of θ_i appearing where estimates of r_i 'ought' to appear. Thus

$$
\begin{aligned}
MSE(\hat{\psi}_N) &= Bias^2(\hat{\psi}_N) + Var(\hat{\psi}_N) \\
&\approx \left[\log\left\{ \frac{\theta_1/(1-\theta_1)}{\theta_0/(1-\theta_0)} \right\} - \psi \right]^2 + \\
&\quad \frac{1}{n_0\theta_0(1-\theta_0)} + \frac{1}{n_1\theta_1(1-\theta_1)}.
\end{aligned}
\tag{5.6}
$$

Figure 5.1 plots the approximate root-mean-squared error in estimating the log odds-ratio ψ as a function of total sample size $n = n_0 + n_1$, assuming $n_0 = n_1$. Plots are given for each of the four combinations of (r_0, r_1, p, q) values studied above. The ideal, adjusted, and naive analyses are considered, so the square roots of (5.4), (5.5), and (5.6) are plotted. As one expects, the error arising from the ideal analysis is usually smaller than that of the adjusted and naive analyses, although in scenarios (iii) and (iv) $MSE(\hat{\psi}_N)$ is slightly smaller than $MSE(\hat{\psi}_I)$ at small sample sizes. Of course $\hat{\psi}_N$ involves an asymptotic bias, whereas $\hat{\psi}_A$ and $\hat{\psi}_I$ do not. Thus for any underlying value of (r_0, r_1, p, q) the naive estimator must be the worst of the three estimators at a large enough sample size. What is surprising, however, is that the sample size may have to be extremely large before the adjusted analysis has a lower MSE than the naive analysis. This is certainly the situation in scenarios (iii) and (iv).

In the narrow sense of bias-variance tradeoff then, the reduction in bias achieved by adjusting for misclassification may not fully offset the increased variability incurred by admitting that misclassification is present. However, this should not be viewed as a justification for using a naive rather than adjusted analysis. In particular, as it is based on a correct model, the adjusted analysis will yield credible intervals for the unknown parameters that achieve the nominal coverage probability asymptotically. In general we expect interval estimates generated via the naive analysis to exhibit undercoverage, given that an incorrect model is being used.

5.2 Partial Knowledge of Misclassification Probabilities

Of course the statistical model described in the previous section presumes that the sensitivity and specificity of the exposure assessment are known. This is likely to be unrealistic in many situations. More realistically, an investigator might have good guesses or estimates for these quantities, but not be convinced that these guesses are perfect. In such an instance the most obvious strategy would be to proceed as before, with the best guesses for the sensitivity and specificity substituted in place of the actual but unknown values. That is, one pretends that the best guesses are exactly correct. While this approach is

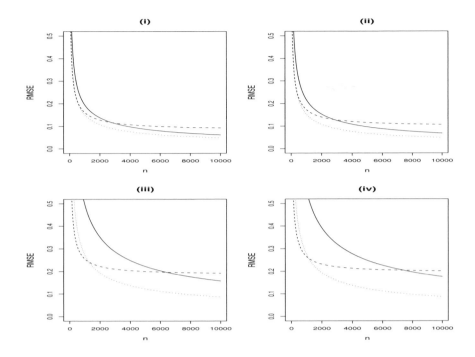

Figure 5.2 *Approximate MSE versus total sample size n for scenarios (i) through (iv). These scenarios underlie datasets (i) through (iv) considered in Table 5.1. In each scenario, the dotted curve corresponds to the ideal posterior, the solid curve to the adjusted posterior, and the dashed curve to the naive posterior.*

formally wrong, one might hope that some robustness obtains. In particular, one might speculate that if the guessed and actual classification probabilities are close to one another, then the corresponding posterior distributions of the log odds-ratio ψ will also be close to one another. Unfortunately, however, Gustafson, Le and Saskin (2001) show that such robustness need not obtain. In particular, they establish the following result.

Let $g(\,\cdot\,;p,q)$ be the function giving apparent exposure prevalences as a function of actual exposure prevalences for given sensitivity p and specificity q. That is, following (5.2),

$$g\left(\left(\begin{array}{c} r_0 \\ r_1 \end{array}\right);p,q\right) = \left(\begin{array}{c} r_0 p + (1 - r_0)(1 - q) \\ r_1 p + (1 - r_1)(1 - q) \end{array}\right).$$

Let (p,q) denote the actual sensitivity and specificity of the exposure assessment, and let (p^*,q^*) be the guessed sensitivity and specificity. Let Ψ be the actual odds-ratio, and let Ψ^* be the large-sample limit of the estimated odds-ratio if the analysis of Section 5.1 is applied with the incorrect values (p^*,q^*).

That is,

$$\Psi^* = \frac{r_1^*/(1-r_1^*)}{r_0^*/(1-r_0^*)},$$

where $r^* = (r_0^*, r_1^*)$ are the incorrectly inferred prevalences of actual exposure $r = (r_0, r_1)$ based on the incorrectly assumed values (p^*, q^*). Specifically,

$$r^* = g^{-1}(g(r; p, q); p^*, q^*). \tag{5.7}$$

Using (5.7), some algebraic manipulation leads to

$$\frac{\Psi^*}{\Psi} = \frac{\{1 + d/r_1\}/\{1 + c/(1 - r_1)\}}{\{1 + d/r_0\}/\{1 + c/(1 - r_0)\}}, \tag{5.8}$$

where $c = (p^* - p)/(p + q - 1)$ and $d = (q^* - q)/(p + q - 1)$. Note that the magnitudes of c and d reflect how close the guessed values are to the actual values. Note also that for any values of c and d, no matter how small, the ratio (5.8) can take on values from zero to infinity as the underlying prevalences (r_0, r_1) vary. This is the essence of the lack of robustness alluded to above. Arbitrarily small discrepancies between the guessed and actual classification probabilities can produce an arbitrarily large bias in the estimated odds-ratio, should the underlying prevalences of exposure happen to be 'unfavourable.'

If the guessed sensitivity and specificity are both overestimates, so that c and d are positive, then (5.8) approaches zero or infinity only when one of the prevalences r_0 or r_1 approaches zero or one. This is a minor comfort, as typically studies are not implemented for exposures with prevalences very close to zero or one. The situation is slightly worse, however, if one or both of the guessed values are underestimates. For instance, if d is negative than (5.8) goes to zero as r_1 decreases to $|d|$, and goes to infinity as r_0 decreases to $|d|$. Thus the difference between Ψ^* and Ψ can become arbitrarily large without the underlying exposure prevalences going to zero or one. In all, the form of (5.8) certainly speaks to a lack of inferential robustness when the assumed values of the sensitivity and specificity differ slightly from the actual values.

As an aside, (5.8) also reveals that discrepancies between the assumed and actual sensitivity and specificity can possibly lead one to infer a nonsensical negative odds-ratio. For instance, say $c > 0$, $d < 0$, $r_0 < |d|$, $r_1 > |d|$. It is clear that (5.8) is negative under these conditions. In fact this can be regarded as useful, as the nonsensical inference alerts the investigator to the fact that the assumed values of (p, q) must be incorrect. In reality, however, the situation is not this clear-cut. For a real sample say $\hat{\theta} = (\hat{\theta}_0, \hat{\theta}_1)$ are the sample proportions of apparent exposure. Then an estimate of Ψ based on estimated prevalences of the form $g^{-1}(\hat{\theta}; p^*, q^*)$ could be negative. However, this would only suggest, and not prove, that (p^*, q^*) are erroneous values. In fact, sampling error in estimating θ by $\hat{\theta}$ can cause $g^{-1}(\hat{\theta}; p, q)$ to yield the same problem even if the correct p and q are used. For the Bayes analysis of Section 5.1 the posterior distribution of θ involves truncation to the interval from $l(p^*, q^*)$ to $r(p^*, q^*)$, which by construction ensures that the posterior distribution on Ψ is restricted to positive values. However, a signal that (p^*, q^*) are wrong may arise if this truncation is excluding values of θ which would otherwise receive appreciable posterior weight.

More generally, Gustafson, Le and Saskin (2001) define the notion of *asymptotically detectable miscorrection* to describe scenarios where one or both of the apparent prevalences (θ_0, θ_1) do *not* lie between $1 - q^*$ and p^*. Since by definition the apparent prevalences must lie between $1 - q$ and p, if the data support one or both apparent prevalences falling outside $(1 - q^*, p^*)$, then the data equally support the notion that the guessed values (p^*, q^*) differ from the actual values (p, q). It is easy to check that a negative value of (5.8) implies an asymptotically detectable miscorrection, though asymptotically detectable miscorrection does not necessarily imply a negative value of (5.8). Gustafson, Le and Saskin (2001) emphasize that the lack of robustness exhibited in (5.8) is still manifested if scenarios involving asymptotically detectable miscorrection are ruled out. Roughly put, one can obtain arbitrarily wrong answers from arbitrarily good guesses for p and q, without this error being detectable from the observed data.

Having suggested that treating good guesses for (p, q) as if they are exact can be problematic, we now consider the alternate strategy of treating (p, q) as unknown parameters. In particular, prior distributions for (p, q) could be centred at the guessed values (p^*, q^*), with the variation in these distributions taken to reflect the investigator's beliefs about the precision of these guesses. Thus we have two possible strategies for analysis which adjusts for the misclassification. For the sake of clarity we distinguish between them as follows. Pretending the guessed values are exact is referred to as *adjusting with false certainty* (AWFC), while assigning priors centred at the guessed values is referred to as *adjusting with uncertainty* (AWU).

The AWU approach to inference is particularly simple if the four unknown parameters (r_0, r_1, p, q) are considered to be independent *a priori*, with prior distributions

$$
\begin{aligned}
r_0 &\sim Unif(0, 1), \\
r_1 &\sim Unif(0, 1), \\
p &\sim Beta(\alpha_p, \beta_p), \\
q &\sim Beta(\alpha_q, \beta_q).
\end{aligned}
$$

In particular we are contemplating situations where the Beta prior distributions for p and q are fairly peaked, as the investigator may have a reasonable idea about how well the exposure assessment performs. On the other hand, one may want to be objective about r_0 and r_1, particularly if the odds-ratio comparing the two prevalences is the parameter of inferential interest. We note that in this framework one could also assign uniform prior distributions to p and q, by setting $\alpha_p = \beta_p = \alpha_q = \beta_q = 1$. However, the model is nonidentifiable, and it seems impossible to generate reasonable inferences with a nonidentifiable model and flat priors for all the parameters. A more focussed discussion of identifiability is given in Section 6.3, but for now we simply note that the model could be reparameterized with $(\theta_0, \theta_1, p, q)$ rather than

(r_0, r_1, p, q) as the unknown parameters, where, as before, (r_0, r_1) are the actual exposure prevalences and (θ_0, θ_1) are the apparent exposure prevalences. This bring the nonidentifiability to the fore, as with the second parameterization the distribution of the data given all the parameters in fact depends only on (θ_0, θ_1), and not on (p, q).

On first glance MCMC fitting of the AWU model would appear to be extremely straightforward. If one works with the original (r_0, r_1, p, q) parameterization and augments the parameter space to include the true but unobserved exposure status of each subject, then all posterior full conditional distributions are standard distributions. Thus it is trivial to implement Gibbs sampling. The details are given in Section 5.6.1. In turns out, however, that the Gibbs sampler does not work well for all datasets in the present context. In a different context Gelfand and Sahu (1999) report poor mixing of the Gibbs sampler for posterior distributions arising from nonidentifiable models, and we have found this to be a problem here as well. Thus Section 5.6.2 describes an alternate MCMC algorithm developed for the AWU model by Gustafson, Le and Saskin (2001). This algorithm operates with the $(\theta_0, \theta_1, p, q)$ parameterization where the lack of identifiability is clearer, and it does *not* augment the parameter space with the true but unobserved exposure status of the study subjects. Specifically, this algorithm is tailored to take advantage of the fact that (θ_0, θ_1) are identified parameters while (p, q) are not. In Section 5.6.3 we demonstrate that for some synthetic data sets the alternate algorithm works quite well while the Gibbs sampler works quite poorly.

The merits of the AWU model compared to the AWFC model are investigated by way of an example with synthetic data. Say that in the context at hand the investigator's best guess for the sensitivity of the exposure assessment is $p^* = 0.9$, and furthermore he is quite confident that the sensitivity is at least 0.8. Thus he assigns p the Beta distribution which has its mode at 0.9 and gives probability 0.9 to the interval $(0.8, 1)$. This determines $p \sim Beta(29.3, 4.1)$. Also, say the investigator's best assessment is that false positives do not arise in the exposure assessment, so that $q^* = 1$. However, he is not certain of this fact. Therefore he takes the prior density for q to have its mode (with finite density) at one, with probability 0.9 assigned to the interval $q \in (0.95, 1)$. This leads to $q \sim Beta(44.9, 1)$. In fact, this argument leading to this particular prior specification was employed by Gustafson, Le and Saskin (2001) in a real scenario where the investigators were uncertain about the assessment of loss of heterozygosity in a cancer case-control study. The two prior densities appear in the first panel of Figure 5.3.

Now say that unbeknownst to the investigators the true sensitivity and specificity of the exposure assessment are $p = 0.85$ and $q = 0.95$. With respect to these actual values, the specified prior distributions are perhaps of 'typical' quality. That is, Figure 5.3 shows that in both cases the actual value lies in the flank of the prior distribution, rather than near the mode or in the tail. Also, say the true exposure prevalences are $r_0 = 0.05$ and $r_1 = 0.0798$, so that $\psi = 0.5$ is the true log odds-ratio. Under these true values of (r_0, r_1, p, q) synthetic data sets are simulated for three sample sizes. For $n_0 = n_1 = 250$ we obtain 15/250 and 33/250 apparent exposures in the control and case samples respectively. Samples that are bigger by a factor of four yield 90/1000 and 113/1000 apparent exposures, while samples that are four times larger again give 366/4000 and 430/4000 apparent exposures.

For each synthetic dataset three posterior distributions for ψ appear in Figure 5.3. The AWU posterior results from the specified prior distributions, while the AWFC posterior is based on the assumption that $(p, q) = (p^*, q^*)$. For the sake of comparison we also present posterior distributions arising if the true values of (p, q) are known. This is referred to as *adjusting with correct certainty* (AWCC). That is, the method of Section 5.1 is applied using the correct values of the sensitivity and specificity. Of course the AWCC posterior distributions are included for the sake of comparison only, as we are interested in real scenarios where the correct values are not known.

A first comment about the posterior distributions is that for identifiable statistical models we expect to see inferences which are twice as precise if the sample size is quadrupled. Indeed, this sort of narrowing with sample size is manifested by the AWFC and AWCC posterior distributions, regardless of the fact that the former posterior distribution is based on an incorrect statistical model, while the latter is based on a correct model. For the nonidentifiable AWU model we do see roughly a factor of two improvement in precision going from $n_j = 250$ to $n_j = 1000$; however the further improvement in going from $n_j = 1000$ to $n_j = 4000$ is much more modest. The large-sample behaviour of posterior distributions arising from nonidentifiable models is considered more closely in Section 6.3.

Figure 5.3 indicates that at all three sample sizes the AWU posterior distribution is better than the AWFC posterior distribution in the sense of being closer to the AWCC posterior distribution. Thus there seems to be a benefit to admitting uncertainty about the sensitivity and specificity via a prior distribution rather than simply pretending that the guessed values of these quantities are correct. More specifically, the AWU posterior distributions tend to be only slightly wider than their AWC counterparts, but importantly this extra width is obtained by extending to the right rather than to the left. In particular, at the largest sample size this extension allows the AWU posterior to cover the true value of $\psi = 0.5$ which is missed by the AWFC posterior.

Of course Figure 5.3 describes inferences arising for particular true values of the parameters (r_0, r_1, p, q). A small simulation study is performed to assess whether there is a general benefit in adjusting with uncertainty compared to adjusting with certainty. We retain the prior distributions described above; that is, $r_0 \sim Unif(0, 1)$, $r_1 \sim Unif(0, 1)$, $p \sim Beta(29.3, 4.1)$, $q \sim Beta(44.9, 1)$. But now we consider average performance when each synthetic dataset is constructed by first simulating values of (p, q, r_0, r_1) from this prior distribution, and then simulating data summaries (S_0, S_1) given (p, q, r_0, r_1). Technically speaking, by examining the average performance of an estimator on repeated synthetic datasets where the true underlying parameters vary from dataset to dataset we are quantifying the Bayes performance of the estimator.

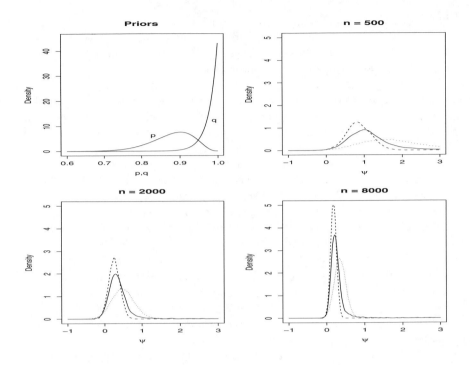

Figure 5.3 *Prior distributions for (p,q) and posterior distributions for ψ in the synthetic data example of Section 5.2. At each sample size the AWFC posterior density (dashed curve), the AWU posterior density (solid curve), and the AWCC posterior density (dotted curve) are given.*

For each synthetic dataset the posterior mean and equal-tailed 80% credible interval for ψ are computed, for each of the AWFC, AWU, and AWCC posterior distributions. These point and interval estimates are then compared to the true value of ψ, bearing in mind that this true value changes with each repetition in the simulation study. Table 5.2 summarizes the results based on 400 synthetic datasets, in terms of the root-mean-squared error of the point estimate, and the coverage probability and average length of the interval estimate.

Table 5.2 shows that the benefit of adjusting with uncertainty over adjusting with false certainty persists more generally, both in terms of smaller $RMSE$ for the point estimate and closer to nominal coverage for the interval estimate. We should point out that both the AWU and $AWCC$ credible intervals are in fact guaranteed to have actual coverage probabilities equal to their nominal coverage probabilities when the underlying parameter values are repeatedly sampled from the prior distribution. In particular, this fundamental property is entirely unaffected by whether the model is identifiable or not. While the $AWFC$ credible intervals tend, on average, to be only half as

	AWFC	AWU	AWCC
RMSE	0.83	0.74	0.45
Coverage	51%	78%	79%
Avg. Length	0.49	0.95	0.64

Table 5.2 *Bayes performance of the adjusted with false certainty (UWFC), adjusted with uncertainty (AWU), and adjusted with correct certainty (AWCC) analyses. The reported results are based on 400 simulated datasets, with the true parameters repeatedly sampled from their prior distribution. The RMSE of the posterior mean and the empirical coverage probability and average length of the 80% equal-tailed credible interval are reported. Note that with 400 repetitions the reported empirical coverage probability will have a simulation standard error of 0.02 if the procedure has an actual coverage probability equal to the nominal 0.8.*

wide as the *AWU* intervals, the low actual coverage probability indicates that this narrowness is neither justified nor desirable.

5.3 Dual Exposure Assessment

Section 5.1 focussed on treating the sensitivity and specificity of the exposure assessment as known, while Section 5.2 considered assigning highly informative priors to these quantities. It may be possible and desirable to avoid both of these approaches, if two different techniques can be used to assess exposure. Such a strategy is fairly common in epidemiological studies. For instance, Hui and Walter (1980) give an example where the exposure of interest is the presence of tuberculosis, with two different diagnostic tests, the Mantoux test and the Tine test, being applied to study subjects. In a case-control study of sudden infant death syndrome, Drews, Flanders and Kosinski (1993) use patient interviews and medical records to provide two assessments of whether subjects are 'exposed' to various putative binary risk factors. Joseph, Gyorkos and Coupal (1995) consider a study in which both a serology test and stool examination are used to test for a particular parasitic infection. And, in a somewhat more complicated setting, Iversen, Parmigiani and Berry (1999) consider a lab test and a family history 'test' for genetic susceptibility to breast cancer.

Letting V again be the actual but unobserved binary exposure variable, V_1^* and V_2^* are used to denote the two imperfect surrogates for V arising from the two assessment schemes. Initially the utility of having two exposure assessments rather than one may not be so clear. It is not reasonable to view V_1^* and V_2^* as replicates or repeated measurements, as generally the distribution of $V_1^*|V$ may be quite different from that of $V_2^*|V$. For instance, one scheme may be much better than the other in the sense of having considerably higher sensitivity and specificity, although this might not be known to the investigator.

Again we consider the retrospective case-control context. Let $c[0, j, k]$ be the number of the n_0 controls for whom $(V_1^* = j, V_2^* = k)$, and let $c[1, j, k]$ be the number of the n_1 cases with these (V_1^*, V_2^*) values. Also, let p_i and q_i be the sensitivity and the specificity of the i-th assessment scheme, for $i = 1, 2$. For now we assume that the two surrogate variables V_1^* and V_2^* are conditionally independent given the actual exposure variable V. This can be interpreted as an assumption about the 'separateness' of the two exposure assessments. In fact it is a strong assumption which is not warranted in all situations, a point we return to later in this section. Given the assumption, the likelihood function for the six unknown parameters takes the form

$$L(p_1, p_2, q_1, q_2, r_0, r_1) = \prod_{j=0}^{1} \prod_{k=0}^{1} \theta_{0jk}^{c[0,j,k]} \theta_{1jk}^{c[1,j,k]}, \qquad (5.9)$$

$$\underbrace{\phantom{\theta_{0jk}^{c[0,j,k]}}}_{\text{controls}} \underbrace{\phantom{\theta_{1jk}^{c[1,j,k]}}}_{\text{cases}}$$

where

$$\theta_{ijk} = \underbrace{r_i}_{\text{exposure prevalence}} p_1^j (1-p_1)^{1-j} p_2^k (1-p_2)^{1-k} +$$
$$(1 - r_i)(1 - q_1)^j q_1^{1-j} (1 - q_2)^k q_2^{1-k} \qquad (5.10)$$

is the probability of observing $(V_1^* = j, V_2^* = k)$ for an individual sampled from the i-th population, i.e., $i = 0$ for controls and $i = 1$ for cases. The form of (5.10) implies that the likelihood function (5.9) depends on its arguments in a complicated manner. As is often the case, however, Bayes-MCMC fitting of this model is greatly simplified by including each subject's true but unobserved exposure variable V as arguments of the posterior distribution. In particular, if the six unknown parameters are assigned independent Beta prior distributions, then all parameters and unobserved variables can be updated simply via Gibbs sampling. Details are given by Johnson, Gastwirth and Pearson (2001).

Initially it seems remarkable to expect good inferences without either external knowledge about the performance of at least one assessment scheme, or gold-standard measurements for at least some study subjects. However, Hui and Walter (1980) illustrate that subject to some minor caveats the model under consideration is identifiable, and therefore consistent estimators of the parameters can be obtained. That is, as more data accumulate, estimates of all the parameters will converge to the corresponding true values. The intuitive argument for identifiability is as follows. Since the data can be summarized in the form of two 2×2 tables, based on the possible (V_1^*, V_2^*) values for controls and cases respectively, we expect to be able to estimate three parameters from each table, or six in total. Since there are in fact six unknown parameters as the arguments for (5.9), it is plausible that they can all be estimated consistently. Indeed, both Hui and Walter (1980) and Drews, Flanders and Kosinski (1993) discuss maximum likelihood estimation for this model. To be more specific, let

$$\phi = (p_1, p_2, q_1, q_2, r_0, r_1)$$

denote the vector of six unknown parameters, and, with reference to (5.10), let

$$\theta = (\theta_{000}, \theta_{001}, \theta_{010}, \theta_{100}, \theta_{101}, \theta_{110}).$$

Note, in particular, that θ completely determines the conditional distribution of $(V_1^*, V_2^*|V)$, as the omitted probabilities θ_{011} and θ_{111} are both deterministic functions of θ, given that the probabilities associated with the conditional distribution must sum to one for both $V = 0$ and $V = 1$. Of course θ can be viewed as a function of ϕ, so we can write $\theta = g(\phi)$, with the form of $g()$ determined by (5.10). Hui and Walter (1980) demonstrate that $g(\cdot)$ is an invertible function, and give an expression, albeit an extremely complicated one, for $g^{-1}(\cdot)$. Thus in principle one can simply estimate θ by cell proportions in the two 2×2 tables which summarize the data. Then, armed with the estimate $\hat{\theta}$, one can estimate ϕ by $\hat{\phi} = g^{-1}(\hat{\theta})$.

Outwardly, the idea that dual exposure assessment can lead to good estimates without having to quantify knowledge about the sensitivity and specificity of the assessments is quite appealing. There are, however, a number of reasons why this should not be viewed as a 'free lunch.' We have already mentioned that the requisite conditional independence assumption may be dubious in specific applications, and indeed we will look more closely at this later in this section. But there are other concerns above and beyond this issue.

An initial concern about this approach to inference is that strictly speaking the function $g(\cdot)$ is two-to-one, so that two distinct ϕ vectors correspond to the observed cell proportions $\hat{\theta}$. Particularly, it is easy to verify from (5.10) that θ is unchanged if we replace each p_i with $1 - q_i$, each q_i with $1 - p_i$, and each r_i with $1 - r_i$. A simple and reasonable solution to this problem is to restrict the parameter space for ϕ according to $p_i + q_i > 1$ for $i = 1, 2$. Clearly an assessment scheme for which $p_i + q_i < 1$ is worse than guessing, and can be ruled out *a priori* in almost any realistic scenario. On the restricted parameter space $g(\cdot)$ is one-to-one, so that $g^{-1}(\cdot)$ is well defined, and $\hat{\phi}$ can be obtained from $\hat{\theta}$.

two population with same prevalence

A second caveat is that the inversion of $g(\cdot)$ breaks down when $r_0 = r_1$. That is, if $r_0 = r_1$ then ϕ cannot be determined from θ. At face value this may not seem worrisome, as it hard to imagine that r_0 and r_1 would be *exactly* the same in any realistic populations of interest. However, as emphasized by Gustafson (2002b), an implication of inference being 'impossible' when $r_0 = r_1$ is that estimators can perform very poorly if r_0 is close to r_1, even at very large sample sizes. In particular, the Fisher information matrix $I(\phi)$ is singular when $r_0 = r_1$, so that the asymptotic variance of estimators of ϕ diverges to infinity as r_0 and r_1 tend toward one another. Indeed, Gustafson (2002b) shows that $|r_0 - r_1|$ need not be very small before the variance of estimators is very large. This is a particular problem in the case-control context, as typically it is not known *a priori* that $|r_0 - r_1|$ will be large.

A third caveat is that sampling variability and/or model misspecification (violation of the conditional independence assumption in particular) can lead to cell probability estimates of θ which actually fall outside the parameter space. That is, $\hat{\theta}$ can lie outside the image under $g(\cdot)$ of the parameter space for ϕ. In such a dataset one cannot obtain an estimate of ϕ of the form $g^{-1}(\hat{\theta})$. Indeed, this problem motivates the work of Drews, Flanders and Kosinski

(1993) who use the EM algorithm to obtain maximum likelihood estimates of ϕ. In particular, they regard the true but unobserved exposure status of each subject as 'missing' data. This approach to maximum likelihood estimation is similar in flavour to the use of Gibbs sampling on an extended parameter space which included the true exposure variables, as described by Johnson, Gastwirth and Pearson (2001).

Bearing these concerns in mind, if one does not want to incorporate any substantive prior information about the parameters it seems reasonable to assign a uniform prior to ϕ, restricted to the region for which $p_i + q_i > 1$ for $i = 1, 2$. The restriction on the parameter space does not cause particular difficulties for Gibbs sampling, as the full conditional posterior distributions for each p_i and q_i become truncated beta distributions rather than beta distributions. However, while the Gibbs sampler is easy to implement, we find it necessary to monitor its output carefully. The MCMC mixing performance can vary considerably across different data sets. Particularly we have noticed poorer mixing for data sets which do not strongly rule out the troublesome $r_0 = r_1$ scenario mentioned above. We describe the results of fitting the model to data shortly, after describing an extension of the model which relaxes the conditional independence assumption.

5.3.1 Relaxing the Conditional Independence Assumption

The assumption that V_1^* and V_2^* are conditionally independent given V may be quite dubious in some applications (Fryback 1978, Brenner 1996, Vacek 1985). Indeed, it is easy to imagine scenarios whereby a subject who is particularly susceptible to misclassification under one assessment scheme is also particularly susceptible under the other scheme. Moreover, the assumption is not empirically verifiable without any gold-standard measurements, as all the 'degrees of freedom' are used to estimate the six unknown parameters. In light of this, Torrance-Rynard and Walter (1997) use simulation to assess the bias introduced by incorrectly assuming the two exposure assessments are conditionally independent given the true exposure. Their findings are mixed, but scenarios where the bias is considerable are given.

We consider extending the model to allow for conditional dependence between V_1^* and V_2^* given V. It is clear, however, that after relaxing the assumption we will no longer have an identifiable model. That is, the data are still summarized in two 2×2 tables, so no more than six parameters can be estimated consistently. However, allowing an unspecified amount of dependence between V_1^* and V_2^* given V clearly increases the number of unknown parameters beyond six. Nonetheless, we investigate such an extension in the face of prior information which reflects the possibility of limited dependence between the two assessments. At the same time we refer the reader ahead to Section 6.3, where some general discussion on the utility of nonidentifiable models is given.

The expanded model postulates that the distribution of (V_1^*, V_2^*) given V depends on six unknown parameters, $(p_1, p_2, q_1, q_2, \delta_0, \delta_1)$, with the form of

		$V_2^* = 0$	$V_2^* = 1$
$V = 0$	$V_1^* = 0$	$q_1 q_2 + \delta_0$	$q_1(1 - q_2) - \delta_0$
	$V_1^* = 1$	$(1 - q_1)q_2 - \delta_0$	$(1 - q_1)(1 - q_2) + \delta_0$

		$V_2^* = 0$	$V_2^* = 1$
$V = 1$	$V_1^* = 0$	$(1 - p_1)(1 - p_2) + \delta_1$	$(1 - p_1)p_2 - \delta_1$
	$V_1^* = 1$	$p_1(1 - p_2) - \delta_1$	$p_1 p_2 + \delta_1$

Table 5.3 *The probabilities describing the conditional distribution of $V_1^*, V_2^* | V$ under the model of Section 5.3.1.*

the distribution given in Table 5.3. It is easy to check that this formulation implies $p_i = Pr(V_i^* = 1 | V = 1)$ and $q_i = Pr(V_i^* = 0 | V = 0)$ for $i = 1, 2$. That is, p_i and q_i retain their interpretation as the sensitivity and specificity of the i-th assessment. As well it is simple to verify that

$$\delta_i = Cov(V_1^*, V_2^* | V = i),$$

so that (δ_0, δ_1) describe the extent to which V_1^* and V_2^* are dependent given V. It is also clear that the observed data in the retrospective study are governed by cell probabilities

$$\theta_{ijk} = r_i \left\{ p_1^j (1 - p_1)^{1-j} p_2^k (1 - p_2)^{1-k} + (-1)^{|j-k|} \delta_1 \right\} +$$
$$(1 - r_i) \left\{ (1 - q_1)^j q_1^{1-j} (1 - q_2)^k q_2^{1-k} + (-1)^{|j-k|} \delta_0 \right\}, \quad (5.11)$$

which generalizes (5.10) as the probability of observing $(V_1^* = j, V_2^* = k)$ for a subject sampled from the i-th population. The probabilities (5.11) yield a likelihood function for the eight unknown parameters, just as (5.10) leads to the likelihood function (5.9) in the model assuming conditional independence.

In terms of a prior we retain the uniform prior for $\phi = (p_1, p_2, q_1, q_2, r_0, r_1)$ over the appropriately restricted parameter space. Then we consider what might be reasonable as a prior for $(\delta_0, \delta_1 | \phi)$. As it is hard to imagine scenarios under which the two surrogates exhibit negative dependence given the true exposure, we use a prior which gives weight only to nonnegative values of δ_0 and δ_1. As well, we must be aware that a legitimate probability distribution for $(V_1^*, V_2^* | V)$ requires

$$\delta_0 \leq \delta_*(q_1, q_2),$$
$$\delta_1 \leq \delta_*(p_1, p_2),$$

where

$$\delta_*(a, b) = \min(a, b) - ab$$

is the maximum possible covariance between two binary random variables with success probabilities a and b. That is, a violation of either inequality corresponds to having at least one entry in Table 5.3 which lies outside the interval from zero to one.

As a further consideration, dependence is inherently more interpretable when expressed in terms of correlation rather than covariance. Thus we define

$$
\begin{aligned}
\rho_0 &= \mathrm{Cor}(V_1^*, V_2^* | V = 0) \\
&= \frac{\delta_0}{\{p_1(1 - p_1)p_2(1 - p_2)\}^{1/2}},
\end{aligned}
$$

and

$$
\begin{aligned}
\rho_1 &= \mathrm{Cor}(V_1^*, V_2^* | V = 1) \\
&= \frac{\delta_1}{\{q_1(1 - q_1)q_2(1 - q_2)\}^{1/2}}.
\end{aligned}
$$

On the one hand it is easier to think about the magnitude of dependence in terms of (ρ_0, ρ_1), but on the other hand the cell probabilities (5.11) are more easily expressed in terms of (δ_0, δ_1).

Given these considerations, we specify a prior density of the form

$$
f(\delta_0, \delta_1 | p_1, p_2, q_1, q_2) = f(\delta_0 | q_1, q_2) f(\delta_1 | p_1, p_2),
$$

with

$$
f(\delta_0 | q_1, q_2) = \frac{\lambda(q_1, q_2) \exp\{-\lambda(q_1, q_2)\delta_0\} I_{[0, \delta_*(q_1, q_2)]}(\delta_0)}{1 - \exp\{-\lambda(q_1, q_2)\delta_*(q_1, q_2)\}}
$$

and

$$
f(\delta_1 | p_1, p_2) = \frac{\lambda(p_1, p_2) \exp\{-\lambda(p_1, p_2)\delta_1\} I_{[0, \delta_*(p_1, p_2)]}(\delta_1)}{1 - \exp\{-\lambda(p_1, p_2)\delta_*(p_1, p_2)\}}.
$$

In the above we take

$$
\lambda(a, b) = \frac{k}{\{a(1 - a)b(1 - b)\}^{1/2}}, \tag{5.12}
$$

where k is a hyperparameter that must be specified. While these expressions are cumbersome, they simply describe truncated exponential priors assigned to the covariance parameters (δ_0, δ_1) given the other parameters. The rate parameters in these exponential distributions, as given by (5.12), are chosen to lend a clear interpretation to the prior in terms of correlation rather than covariance. For instance, consider a value $\delta_0 = \tilde{\delta}_0$ which corresponds to a correlation $\rho_0 = \tilde{\rho}_0$. The ratio of the prior density at $\delta_0 = \tilde{\delta}_0$ to the prior density at $\delta_0 = 0$ can be expressed as $\exp(-k\tilde{\rho}_0)$. Thus k can be chosen to reflect the strength of the belief that the conditional dependence is not likely to be strong. In the examples that follow, for instance, we choose $k = 4\log 4$ in the priors for both δ_0 and δ_1. Then the prior downweights $\rho_i = 0.25$ by a factor of four relative to $\rho_i = 0$, for $i = 0, 1$.

As alluded to in Section 5.2, there is some literature to suggest that standard MCMC algorithms do not always perform well on posterior distributions arising from nonidentifiable models. This issue seems particularly germane to

exposure		controls		cases	
		$V_2^* = 0$	$V_2^* = 1$	$V_2^* = 0$	$V_2^* = 1$
anemia	$V_1^* = 0$	147	15	125	15
	$V_1^* = 1$	34	20	49	24
UTI	$V_1^* = 0$	190	4	174	14
	$V_1^* = 1$	10	14	14	13
LWG	$V_1^* = 0$	86	4	73	5
	$V_1^* = 1$	3	6	13	11

Table 5.4 *Data from a SIDS case-control study. Three binary exposures are considered: maternal anemia during pregnancy, maternal urinary tract infection (UTI) during pregnancy, and low weight-gain (LWG) during pregnancy. Each exposure is assessed by maternal interview (V_1^*) and by examination of medical records (V_2^*).*

algorithms which update one parameter at a time using the obvious or original parameterization of the problem. Our experience is that MCMC algorithms can perform poorly when applied to the current model, and in Section 5.6.4 we detail an algorithm designed to ameliorate this problem as much as possible. Particularly, this scheme updates (q_1, q_2, δ_0) and (p_1, p_2, δ_1) in blocks, taking into account the structure depicted in Table 5.3.

5.3.2 Example

For the sake of clarity we henceforth refer to the two dual exposure assessment models described in this section as DUAL-IND and DUAL-DEP, with the former assuming conditional independence of the two assessments and the latter placing a prior distribution on the magnitude of dependence. Both models are applied to data given by Drews, Flanders and Kosinski (1993) from a case-control study on sudden infant death syndrome (SIDS). In the first instance the binary exposure variable is maternal anemia during pregnancy, assessed by both an interview with the mother and an examination of the mother's medical records. Neither method can be considered a gold-standard, and it is immediately apparent from the data summarized in Table 5.4 that the two assessments are in disagreement for a substantial fraction of the study subjects.

The upper-left panel of Figure 5.4 gives the posterior distribution of the log odds-ratio $\psi = log\{r_1/(1 - r_1)\} - log\{r_0/(1 - r_0)\}$ under both the DUAL-IND and DUAL-DEP models. We see that DUAL-DEP yields a wider posterior distribution than DUAL-IND. That is, admitting uncertainty about the dependence leads to more inferential uncertainty *a posteriori*, as one might expect. On the other hand, the posterior mode of ψ is quite similar under the two models. Admitting uncertainty about whether the conditional independence assumption is appropriate does not produce a substantial change in the point estimate of ψ.

For the sake of comparison we also try a third, more naive, modelling strategy. In particular we consider using only the data from those subjects with concordant assessments, i.e., $V_1^* = V_2^*$. The concordant value is then treated as if it is the actual exposure V. We label this strategy as DUAL-CON. From Figure 5.4 we see that the widths of the DUAL-CON and DUAL-IND posterior distributions for ψ are very similar, but the DUAL-CON posterior mode lies somewhat closer to zero than the DUAL-IND or DUAL-DEP posterior modes. This attentuation is not surprising, as to some extent the DUAL-CON strategy is ignoring the misclassification rather than adjusting for it.

Given the lack of identifiability in the DUAL-DEP model, there is concern about how well this model can be fit to data via MCMC methods. The upper-right panel of Figure 5.4 gives a traceplot of the MCMC output for ψ under this model. The mixing behaviour seems tolerable, despite the lack of identifiability. Also, the lower panels of Figure 5.4 give posterior scatterplots of ψ versus ρ_0 and ψ versus ρ_1 under the DUAL-DEP model. We note that the posterior correlations are weak in both cases. In part this explains why DUAL-DEP and DUAL-IND point estimates of ψ are similar, as the posterior distribution of ψ given the dependence parameters does not depend strongly on the dependence parameters.

In fact, Drews, Flanders and Kosinksi (1993) considered various binary exposures in this study. Table 5.4 also gives data for the exposures maternal urinary tract infection during pregnancy and low weight gain during pregnancy. Figures 5.5 and 5.6 summarize the posterior analyses for these exposures, in the same format as Figure 5.4. The qualitative findings for these exposures are very similar to those for the maternal anemia exposure. That is, the DUAL-IND and DUAL-DEP posterior distributions for ψ have modes at very similar values, but the former distribution is much narrower than the latter. In comparison, the DUAL-CON posterior mode is closer to zero. The MCMC mixing for the nonidentifiable DUAL-DEP model is tolerable, and the posterior correlation between ψ and ρ_i is weak, for both $i = 0$ and $i = 1$.

As a whole, experience with the three different exposures suggests that the DUAL-IND modelling strategy may have some robustness, in the sense of yielding similar point estimates of ψ to those under the more general DUAL-DEP model. It is also clear, however, that if an investigator is really unsure about the conditional independence assumption then the DUAL-IND posterior distribution is considerably over-confident, as it tends to be much narrower than its DUAL-DEP counterpart. We have also demonstrated that fitting the DUAL-DEP model, which reflects a prior downweighting of larger correlations between V_1^* and V_2^* given V, is a plausible inferential strategy, even though the model is formally nonidentifiable.

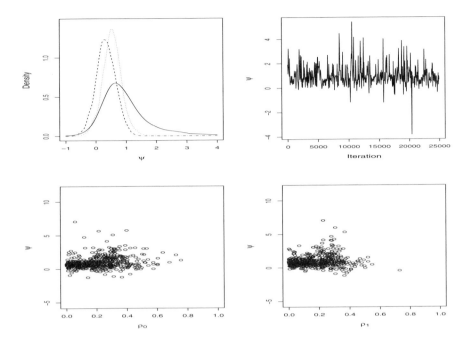

Figure 5.4 *Posterior summaries for the SIDS example, with maternal anemia as the exposure variable. The upper-left panel gives the posterior distribution of the log odds-ratio ψ under the DUAL-IND model (dotted curve), the DUAL-DEP model (solid curve), and the DUAL-CON approach (dashed curve). The upper-right panel gives the MCMC output for ψ under the DUAL-DEP model, while the scatterplots in the lower panels depict the joint posterior distribution of (ρ_0, ψ) and (ρ_1, ψ) under this model.*

5.4 Models with Additional Explanatory Variables

Thus far in this chapter we have examined inferences in the focussed framework of a single binary exposure, with either one or two imperfect assessments of this exposure. Of course many studies involve multiple explanatory variables. In such instances the paradigm of measurement, outcome, and exposure models described in Chapter 4 can be applied equally well to a binary exposure. Consider a random sample of n observations on (V_1^*, V_2^*, Y, Z), where V_1^* and V_2^* are two different surrogates for the actual binary exposure V, Y is the outcome variable, and Z is a vector of precisely measured covariates. A measurement model parameterized by α, an outcome model parameterized by β, and an exposure model parameterized by γ can be combined to yield a posterior distribution

$$f(\alpha, \beta, \gamma, v | v_1^*, v_2^*, y, z) \quad \propto \quad \prod_{i=1}^{n} f(v_{1i}^*, v_{2i}^* | y_i, v_i, z_i, \alpha) \times$$

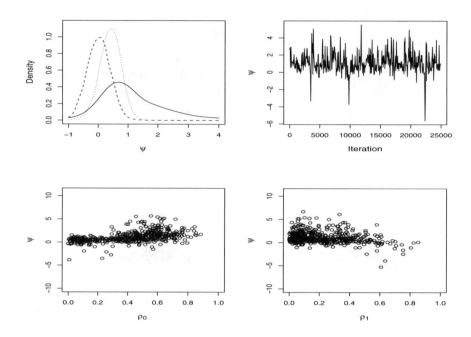

Figure 5.5 *Posterior summaries for the SIDS example, with maternal urinary tract infection as the exposure variable. The format is the same as Figure 5.4.*

$$\prod_{i=1}^{n} f(y_i|v_i, z_i, \beta) \ \times$$

$$\prod_{i=1}^{n} f(v_i|z_i, \gamma) \ \times$$

$$f(\alpha, \beta, \gamma). \tag{5.13}$$

In the case of a binary exposure V, however, this may not be the most pragmatic way to proceed. In particular, the contribution of the outcome and exposure models may be re-expressed as

$$f(y|v, z)f(v|z) \ = \ f(y, v|z)$$
$$= \ f(v|y, z)f(y|z).$$

Thus an alternative strategy is to use what we will call a *exposure given outcome model*, by specifying a distributional form for $V|Y, Z$ parameterized by λ rather than separate outcome and exposure models as in (5.13). Importantly, in doing so it is not necessary to parameterize the distribution of $Y|Z$, as both

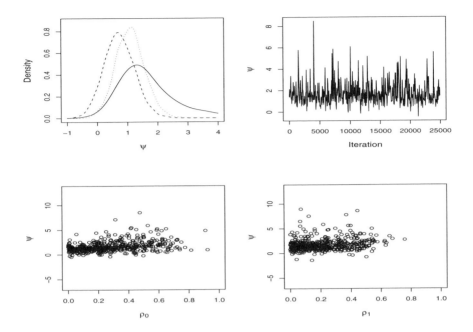

Figure 5.6 *Posterior summaries for the SIDS example, with low pregnancy weight gain as the exposure variable. The format is the same as Figure 5.4.*

Y and Z are observed. Thus we have

$$
\begin{aligned}
f(\alpha, \lambda, v | v_1^*, v_2^*, y, z) \quad &\propto \quad \prod_{i=1}^{n} f(v_{1i}^*, v_{2i}^* | v_i, y_i, z_i, \alpha) \; \times \\
&\quad \prod_{i=1}^{n} f(v_i | y_i, z_i, \lambda) \; \times \\
&\quad f(\alpha, \lambda),
\end{aligned}
\tag{5.14}
$$

where the $f(y|z)$ term can be omitted, since we need only the posterior density of (α, λ, v) up to a constant of proportionality.

The obvious pragmatic advantage of (5.14) over (5.13) is that one need only estimate two parameter vectors rather than three. Moreover, when Y and V are both binary an exposure given outcome model may be just as good at describing the exposure-outcome relationship as is an outcome model. Particularly, standard logistic regression outcome and exposure models would be

$$
\mathrm{logit} \, Pr(Y = 1 | V, Z) \quad = \quad \beta_0 + \beta_1 V + \beta_2' Z,
\tag{5.15}
$$

and

$$\operatorname{logit} Pr(V = 1|Z) \quad = \quad \gamma_0 + \gamma_1' Z. \tag{5.16}$$

Together these define the joint distribution of (Y, V) given Z, and subsequently the conditional distribution of V given (Y, Z). Indeed, straightforward calculation gives

$$\operatorname{logit} Pr(V = 1|Y, Z) \quad = \quad \gamma_0 + \beta_1 Y + \gamma_1' Z + g(Z; \beta), \tag{5.17}$$

where

$$g(z; \beta) \quad = \quad \log \left\{ 1 + \exp(\beta_0 + \beta_2' z) \right\} - \log \left\{ 1 + \exp(\beta_0 + \beta_1 + \beta_2' z) \right\}.$$

In particular, given Z, β_1 has a well-known dual interpretation. Conditioned on any fixed value of Z it is the log odds-ratio for both Y in terms of X and X in terms of Y. In particular, this suggests that using an exposure given outcome model of the form

$$\operatorname{logit} Pr(V = 1|Y, Z) \quad = \quad \lambda_0 + \lambda_1 Y + \lambda_2' Z \tag{5.18}$$

is nearly equivalent to using (5.15) and (5.16), the slight difference being the omission of the nonlinear term $g(Z; \beta)$ in (5.17). Moreover, λ_1 in (5.18) can be interpreted as if it were β_1 in the outcome model (5.15).

We note that in principle one could use an exposure given outcome model instead of separate outcome and exposure models when one or both of V and Y are continuous. This is less attractive, however, as the two approaches will no longer have the similarity and dual interpretation of parameters exhibited in the binary case.

5.4.1 Example

As an example which contrasts the use of an exposure given outcome model with the use of separate outcome and exposure models we consider a dataset presented by Kosinski and Flanders (1999). These data arose from a clinical study of patients with multi-vessel coronary artery disease. The main purpose of the study was to compare two therapies, percutaneous transluminal coronary angioplasty (PTCA) and coronary artery bypass grafting (CABG), with patients randomized to the two therapies. In fact the study did not establish a statistically significant difference between the therapies with respect to the composite primary endpoint. As a secondary issue, Kosinski and Flanders consider whether the presence $(V = 1)$ of haemodynamically obstructive coronary artery disease (HCAD) at a one-year follow up visit after the initial procedure (PTCA or CABG) is associated with the occurrence of a future cardiac event. A future cardiac event $(Y = 1)$ is defined as a subsequent procedure, myocardial infarction, or death between 90 days and 2 years after the follow-up visit.

The HCAD status V cannot be measured without error. The first surrogate V_1^* is based on an exercise stress test. The second surrogate V_2^* is based on a single-photon-emission computed tomography (SPECT) thallium test.

Y	Z_1	Z_2	freq.		$V_2^* = 0$	$V_2^* = 1$
0	0	0	147	$V_1^* = 0$	85	46
				$V_1^* = 1$	10	6
0	0	1	60	$V_1^* = 0$	44	12
				$V_1^* = 1$	1	3
0	1	0	66	$V_1^* = 0$	36	20
				$V_1^* = 1$	3	7
0	1	1	7	$V_1^* = 0$	4	1
				$V_1^* = 1$	1	1
1	0	0	12	$V_1^* = 0$	7	3
				$V_1^* = 1$	0	2
1	0	1	8	$V_1^* = 0$	5	1
				$V_1^* = 1$	0	2
1	1	0	14	$V_1^* = 0$	4	6
				$V_1^* = 1$	2	2
1	1	1	1	$V_1^* = 0$	0	0
				$V_1^* = 1$	0	1

Table 5.5 *Data from Kosinski and Flanders (1999). For each combination of Y (non-occurrence/occurrence of cardiac event), Z_1 (weight less/more than 90 kg), and Z_2 (male/female) the observed V_1^* (surrogate for HCAD based on exercise stress test) and V_2^* (surrogate for HCAD based on SPECT thallium test) values are summarized in a 2×2 table. The total sample size is $n = 315$ subjects.*

It is clear from the data, which are summarized in Table 5.5, that the two surrogates are discrepant for a substantial proportion of the study subjects. Drews and Kosinski consider two binary covariates: weight in comparison to a threshold and gender. In particular, weight (Z_1) is coded as zero/one based on a subject's weight being less/more than 90 kg, while gender (Z_2) is coded as zero/one for male/female.

We apply logistic regression models to these data. In the first instance we use outcome model (5.15) and exposure model (5.16), and in the second instance we instead use the exposure given outcome model (5.18). Either way we assume the misclassification is nondifferential and the two surrogates for exposure are conditionally independent given the true but unobserved exposure. Thus, as previously, the misclassification model involves four unknown parameters, namely the sensitivity p_i and specificity q_i of the i-th exposure assessment, $i = 1, 2$. In all, the first approach involves $4 + 4 + 3 = 13$ unknown parameters, while the second involves $4 + 4 = 8$ unknown parameters. The requisite MCMC analysis is easily implemented under either strategy. Particularly, the MCMC updating schemes for logistic regression models described in Section 4.11 can be applied here quite directly.

Selected posterior distributions are displayed in Figure 5.7. In particular, the posterior distribution of p_1, p_2, q_1, q_2 and the log-odds describing the relationship between Y and V given Z are given for each modelling strategy. Recall that the latter is β_1 in the first model and λ_1 in the second model. For all five parameters of interest the posterior distributions based on the two models are virtually the same. This lends credence to opting for the simpler specification of an exposure given outcome model whenever possible.

5.4.2 Beyond Nondifferential and Conditionally Independent Dual Exposure Assessment

With the DUAL-IND model of Section 5.3 we could not relax the assumption of conditionally independent assessments without losing the identifiability of the model. With the availability of other precisely measured covariates, however, the situation may be improved. Kosinski and Flanders (1999) consider a very general approach with the measurement model specified via two logistic regression models,

$$\text{logit} Pr(V_2^* = 1 | V_1^*, V, Y, Z) = \alpha_0 + \alpha_1 V_1^* + \alpha_2 V + \alpha_3 Y + \alpha_4 Z$$

$$(5.19)$$

and

$$\text{logit} Pr(V_1^* = 1 | V, Y, Z) = \alpha_5 + \alpha_6 V + \alpha_7 Y + \alpha_8 Z, \qquad (5.20)$$

along with a third logistic regression model for the exposure given outcome:

$$\text{logit} Pr(V = 1 | Y, Z) = \lambda_0 + \lambda_1 Y + \lambda_2 Z. \qquad (5.21)$$

Sub-models of this general model then correspond to commonly used models. For instance, the assumption that the misclassification is nondifferential corresponds to $\alpha_3 = \alpha_4 = \alpha_7 = \alpha_8 = 0$, which makes (V_1^*, V_2^*) and (Y, Z) conditionally independent given V. The other obvious sub-model is that arising when $\alpha_1 = 0$, which corresponds to V_1^* and V_2^* being conditionally independent given (V, Y, Z).

The position taken by Kosinski and Flanders (1999) is that one can actually assess how well supported these various models are in light of the data. In some formal sense this will be the case if the full model is identifiable, so that all the unknown parameters in (5.19), (5.20), and (5.21) can be estimated consistently. To consider whether this might be the case, say that Z is comprised of p covariates, all of which are binary. Moreover, say that the joint distribution of (Y, Z) gives positive probability to all 2^{p+1} possible values. Since the data can be summarized in the form of separate 2×2 tables for (V_1^*, V_2^*) values given each combination of (Y, Z) values, we might expect to be able to estimate as many as $3 \times 2^{p+1}$ unknown parameters consistently. Moreover, a

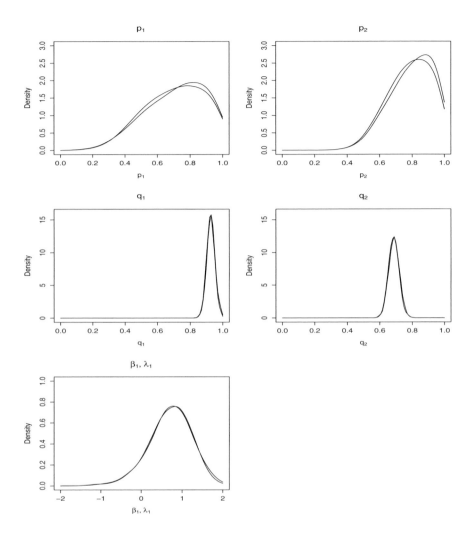

Figure 5.7 *Posterior summaries for the coronary example. Posterior distributions for p_1, p_2, q_1, q_2 and the conditional log odds-ratio for the outcome-exposure relationship (β_1 in the outcome model or λ_1 in the exposure given outcome model) are given, for each of the two models considered.*

quick count reveals a total of $(p + 4) + (p + 3) + (p + 2) = 3p + 9$ unknown parameters in the full model. For $p = 1$, the two totals are equal, and for $p > 1$ the upper bound on the number of consistently estimable parameters exceeds the actual number of unknown parameters. While this counting argument does not *prove* that the full model is identifiable provided there is at least one precisely measured covariate, it does suggest this might be the case.

Kosinski and Flanders (1999) report results from maximum likelihood fitting based on (5.19) through (5.21), without assuming the two exposure assessments are nondifferential and conditionally independent. Specifically, they give results for the HCAD dataset considered in Section 5.4.2 as well as for a simulated dataset. Unfortunately, however, our experience with Bayes-MCMC fitting of the same models is quite discouraging. Even assuming nondifferential misclassification ($\alpha_3 = \alpha_4 = \alpha_7 = \alpha_8 = 0$) but allowing dependence (α_1 unconstrained) is extremely problematic. MCMC algorithms tend to mix poorly, and when applied to synthetic datasets very poor results obtain. In particular, the posterior distribution of α_1 tends to concentrate away from zero even if the data are simulated under $\alpha_1 = 0$.

As an alternative strategy we considered using the measurement model from the DUAL-DEP model described in Section 5.3.1, in tandem with the exposure given outcome model (5.21). This involves two parameters (δ_0, δ_1) which describe the dependence between assessments, rather than the single parameter (α_1) in (5.19) and (5.20). Rather than assign an informative prior to (δ_0, δ_1) as before, we now use a flat prior, given that we have enough 'degrees-of-freedom' to estimate all the unknown parameters. Unfortunately this strategy also yields very poor performance, both in terms of poor MCMC mixing and posterior distributions from synthetic datasets which miss the true values of parameters.

The negative experiences from these modelling strategies suggest it is very difficult to fit models which do not either specify the dependence parameters exactly or at least assign them relatively informative prior distributions. Thus the theoretical gain in degrees of freedom afforded by additional precisely measured explanatory variables does not always translate to a practical ability to fit models entailing fewer assumptions.

5.4.3 Dual Exposure Assessment in Three Populations

To shed more light on the difficulty inherent in relaxing the conditional independence assumption, consider the following situation. Say we can sample surrogate exposures (V_1^*, V_2^*) in three distinct populations having exposure prevalences (r_0, r_1, r_2). Thus we can hope to estimate nine parameters from the observed data. If we do assume nondifferential misclassification but do not assume conditional independence of the two assessments then there are nine unknown parameters. In addition to the three unknown prevalences, the six parameters $(p_1, p_2, q_1, q_2, \delta_0, \delta_1)$ govern the distribution of $(V_1^*, V_2^* | V)$, exactly as in the DUAL-DEP model from Section 5.3.1.

In the case of two populations and two conditionally independent exposure assessments we know that the six unknown parameters can be estimated consistently. However, as illustrated by Gustafson (2002) the variance of the estimators can be extremely large if the two population prevalences are not well-separated. The same problem may persist, or in fact be worse, in the present context of three populations and unknown dependence parameters. Indeed, this may explain the difficulties described at the end of the previous subsection.

To investigate, let $S^{(i)}$ be a vector of length four which summarizes the sampled (V_1^*, V_2^*) values in the sample from the i-th population, for $i = 0, 1, 2$. Formally, $S^{(i)}$ is the sum over the sampled subjects of $V_1^* V_2^*$, $V_1^*(1 - V_2^*)$, $(1 - V_1^*)V_2^*$, and $(1 - V_1^*)(1 - V_2^*)$. That is, $S^{(i)}$ simply comprises the cells of the 2×2 table summarizing the data from the i-th sample. Also, let

$$
\theta = \begin{pmatrix} p_1 p_2 + \delta_1 \\ p_1(1 - p_2) - \delta_1 \\ (1 - p_1)p_2 - \delta_1 \\ (1 - p_1)(1 - p_2) + \delta_1 \end{pmatrix}
$$

be the cell probabilities for a truly exposed subject, while

$$
\phi = \begin{pmatrix} (1 - q_1)(1 - q_2) + \delta_0 \\ (1 - q_1)q_2 - \delta_0 \\ q_1(1 - q_2) - \delta_0 \\ q_1 q_2 + \delta_0 \end{pmatrix}
$$

are the corresponding cell probabilities for a truly unexposed subject.

Clearly the observed data are distributed as

$$
S^{(i)} \sim Multinomial(n_i; r_i \theta + (1 - r_i)\phi).
$$

Now let $Z^{(i)}$ denote the (unobservable) counts for only the truly exposed subjects in the i-th sample. Then

$$
\begin{pmatrix} Z^{(i)} \\ S^{(i)} - Z^{(i)} \end{pmatrix} \sim Multinomial \left(n_i; \begin{pmatrix} r_i \theta \\ (1 - r_i)\phi \end{pmatrix} \right), \tag{5.22}
$$

which we can regard as the distribution of the 'complete' data. Of course in reality only $S^{(i)}$ is observed, but (5.22) is useful for the purposes of MCMC algorithm construction. Indeed, in Section 5.6.5 we outline the straightforward approach to Gibbs sampling in this scenario.

In light of the apparent identifiability in this problem we consider the use of uniform priors on θ, ϕ, r_0, r_1, and r_2. However, to avoid the trivial non-identifiability that arises by interchanging θ and ϕ as well as r_i and $1 - r_i$, we restrict the parameter space according to $\theta_1 > \phi_1$ and $\theta_4 < \phi_4$. That is, the probability of a subject being classified as exposed by both assessments is greater for a truly exposed subject than for a truly unexposed subject, and similarly the probability of a subject being classified as unexposed by both assessments is greater for a truly unexposed subject than for a truly exposed subject.

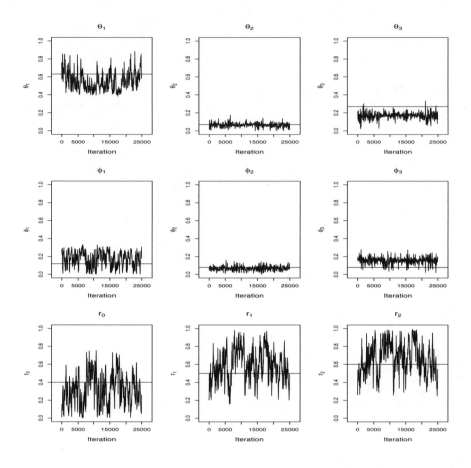

Figure 5.8 *MCMC output for the first synthetic dataset in the three population example of Section 5.4.3. Specifically, 25000 Gibbs sampler iterations are displayed. The superimposed horizontal lines denote true parameter values.*

Three synthetic datasets are generated, each based on $\theta = (.63, .07, .27, .03)$ which corresponds to $p_1 = 0.9$, $p_2 = 0.7$, $\delta_1 = 0$, and $\phi = (.72, .08, .08, .12)$, which corresponds to $q_1 = 0.8$, $q_2 = 0.8$, $\delta_0 = 0.08$. Thus V_1^* and V_2^* are conditionally independent given that $V = 1$, but have a correlation of 0.5 given that $V = 0$.

The first dataset is based on samples of size $n_i = 500$, for $i = 0, 1, 2$, with underlying exposure prevalences of $(r_0, r_1, r_2) = (0.4, 0.5, 0.6)$. MCMC traceplots for the posterior distribution of the parameters given this dataset appear in Figure 5.8. In addition to very poor MCMC mixing, we see the algorithm visiting parameter values very far from the true values. There does not appear to be hope of making reasonable inferences in this scenario.

To see if increased sample sizes lead to reasonable inferences, a larger dataset is simulated under the same parameter values. This time samples of size 2000

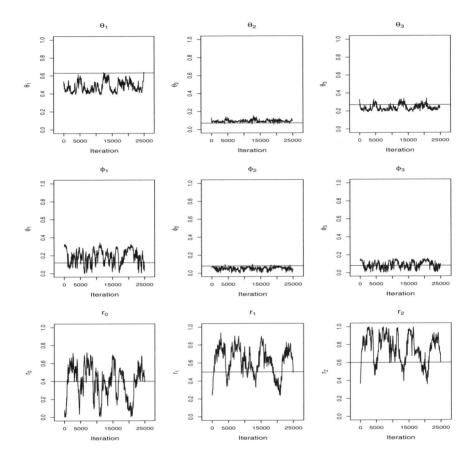

Figure 5.9 *MCMC output for the second synthetic dataset in the three population example of Section 5.4.3. Specifically, 25000 Gibbs sampler iterations are displayed. The superimposed horizontal lines denote true parameter values.*

are drawn from each population, giving a sample size of 6000 in all. The MCMC output based on these data is given in Figure 5.9. Unfortunately we do not see a marked reduction in either statistical error or simulation error. In particular, as best one can tell given the poor mixing, the posterior distribution over the unknown prevalences is very wide.

Given our discussion of the DUAL-IND model in Section 5.3.1, one suspects that the limitations on inference from the second synthetic dataset arise because the underlying exposure prevalences in the three populations are not sufficiently disparate. Thus our third dataset again involves $n_i = 2000$ subjects per population, but now the underlying prevalences are taken to be $(r_0, r_1, r_2) = (0.2, 0.5, 0.8)$. The resultant MCMC output appears in Figure 5.10. While there is some improvement in the MCMC mixing, the posterior distributions over the prevalences are still very wide. Even with a lot of data

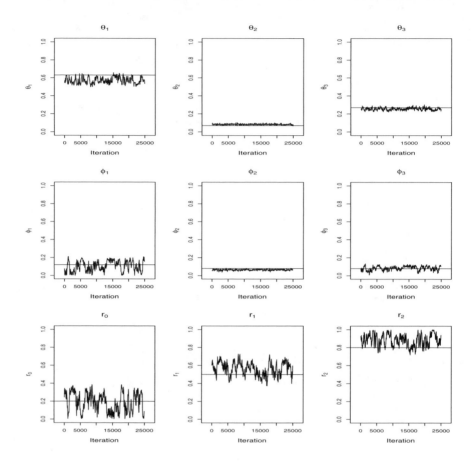

Figure 5.10 *MCMC output for the third synthetic dataset in the three population example of Section 5.4.3. Specifically, 25000 Gibbs sampler iterations are displayed. The superimposed horizontal lines denote true parameter values.*

and *very* disparate prevalences it is difficult to estimate the prevalences with any precision.

We find these results to be quite discouraging with regard to the sort of modelling alluded to at the start of this section. In principle we gain the ability to estimate more parameters when additional precisely measured explanatory variables are available, as each combination of levels of these variables constitutes a population with a distinct exposure prevalence. However, in most practical applications the exposure prevalence will only vary weakly with the covariates and response variable, so one is unlikely to see large differences in prevalences across these populations. And the present findings suggest that good estimation is not possible even with quite substantial variation in prevalence.

5.5 Summary

We have seen that Bayes-MCMC analysis provides a straightforward route to statistical inference which accounts for misclassification of a binary explanatory variable. Roughly speaking, we have considered two routes to obtaining sufficient information for a meaningful analysis to proceed. The first route involves the use of prior information about the misclassification; the second uses dual surrogates for the unobservable variable. We have observed numerous subtleties surrounding the performance of adjusted estimates, and also noted that often something more than 'off-the-shelf' MCMC techniques may be needed for model fitting. Finally, we have seen that simply having a rich enough data structure to potentially estimate the number of parameters at play does not always translate to actual good performance of estimators.

It would be remiss not to mention a number of papers that touch on similar ideas to those exhibited in this chapter. Indeed, a number of authors have considered Bayesian analysis which adjusts for misclassification of categorical variables, though often the focus is not on misclassification in explanatory variables *per se*. Related references include Johnson and Gastwirth (1991), Viana and Ramakrishnan (1992), Viana (1994), Evans, Guttman, Haitovsky, and Swartz (1995), and Tu, Kowalski, and Jia (1999).

5.6 Mathematical Details

5.6.1 Gibbs Sampling for the AWU Model of Section 5.2

The naive Gibbs sampler for fitting the AWU model of Section 5.2 would augment the (r_0, r_1, p, q) parameter space with the actual exposure V for each study subject. We denote the actual and surrogate exposure variables for the i-th subject in the j-th sample as V_{ji} and V_{ji}^* respectively. Clearly the naive Gibbs sampler would involve $n_0 + n_1 + 4$ individual updates at each iteration.

In fact it is more expedient to update sufficient statistics rather than the individual V variables, thereby obtaining an algorithm with an execution time that does not increase with the sample size. If we had complete data, that is observations of both V and V^* for each subject, then sufficient statistics would be (S_0, A_0, B_0) and (S_1, A_1, B_1), where

$$S_j = \sum_{i=1}^{n_j} V_{ji}^*$$

$$A_j = \sum_{i=1}^{n_j} V_{ji} V_{ji}^*$$

$$B_j = \sum_{i=1}^{n_j} (1 - V_{ji})(1 - V_{ji}^*).$$

That is, for sample j, S_j is the total number of apparent exposures, A_j is the total number of simultaneous actual and apparent exposures, and B_j is the total number of simultaneous actual and apparent unexposures. Clearly the distribution of the complete data is given by

$$
\begin{pmatrix} A_j \\ B_j \\ S_j - A_j \\ n_j - S_j - B_j \end{pmatrix} \sim Multinomial \left(n_j; \begin{pmatrix} r_j p \\ (1 - r_j)q \\ (1 - r_j)(1 - q) \\ r_j(1 - p) \end{pmatrix} \right),
$$

$$(5.23)$$

independently for $j = 0, 1$.

From (5.23) and the prior described in Section 5.2 we immediately see the form of the joint posterior density for the unobserved quantities $U = (p, q, r_0, r_1, a_0, a_1, b_0, b_1)$ given the observed quantities $O = (s_0, s_1)$. Specifically,

$$
\begin{aligned}
f(U|O) \quad \propto \quad & \frac{1}{a_0! b_0! (s_0 - a_0)! (n_0 - s_0 - b_0)!} \times \\
& \frac{1}{a_1! b_1! (s_1 - a_1)! (n_1 - s_1 - b_1)!} \times \\
& r_0^{a_0 + n_0 - s_0 - b_0} (1 - r_0)^{b_0 + s_0 - a_0} \times \\
& r_1^{a_1 + n_1 - s_1 - b_1} (1 - r_1)^{b_1 + s_1 - a_1} \times \\
& p^{\alpha_p - 1 + a_0 + a_1} (1 - p)^{\beta_p - 1 + n_0 + n_1 - s_0 - s_1 - b_0 - b_1} \times \\
& q^{\alpha_q - 1 + b_0 + b_1} (1 - q)^{\beta_q - 1 + s_0 + s_1 - a_0 - a_1}.
\end{aligned}
$$

Clearly then the full conditional posterior distribution for each of (r_0, r_1, p, q) is a Beta distribution, with parameters that are easily 'read off' from the expression above. For instance, r_0 given the other unobservables and the observables has a $Beta(1 + a_0 + n_0 - s_0 - b_0, b_0 + s_0 - a_0)$ distribution.

Somewhat closer inspection of the expression for $f(U|O)$ reveals that each of (a_0, b_0, a_1, b_1) has a binomial full conditional posterior distribution. For instance, as a function of a_0 alone the expression is proportional to

$$
\frac{1}{a_0! (s_0 - a_0)!} r_0^{a_0} (1 - r_0)^{-a_0} p^{a_0} (1 - q)^{-a_0},
$$

whence

$$
a_0 | a_0^C \sim Binomial \left(s_0, \frac{r_0 p}{r_0 p + (1 - r_0)(1 - q)} \right),
$$

where a_0^C denotes all the elements of (U, O) except a_0. Thus the Gibbs sampler is easily applied to this model. All that is required is sampling from beta and binomial distributions.

5.6.2 A Tailored MCMC Algorithm for the AWU Model of Section 5.2

As alluded to in Section 5.2, Gibbs sampling is not necessarily an effective MCMC algorithm for nonidentifiable models. Here an alternate algorithm which is tailored to the particular model is presented.

Upon reparameterizing from (r_0, r_1, p, q) to $(\theta_0, \theta_1, p, q)$, the prior distribution formulated with respect to the original parameters becomes

$$f(\theta_0, \theta_1, p, q) \quad \propto \quad \frac{b(p; \alpha_p, \beta_p)b(q; \alpha_q, \beta_q)}{(p+q-1)^2} I_{A(\theta_0,\theta_1)}(p,q), \qquad (5.24)$$

where $b(\cdot, \alpha, \beta)$ denote the Beta density function with parameters (α, β), while

$$A(\theta_0, \theta_1) \quad = \quad \{(p,q) : 0 < p < \underline{\theta}, 0 < q < 1 - \bar{\theta}\} \quad \cup$$
$$\{(p,q) : \bar{\theta} < p < 1, 1 - \underline{\theta} < q < 1\}, \qquad (5.25)$$

with $\underline{\theta} = \min\{\theta_0, \theta_1\}$ and $\bar{\theta} = \max\{\theta_0, \theta_1\}$. Note in particular that the $(p + q - 1)^{-2}$ term in (5.24) arises from the Jacobian associated with the transformation, while the restriction of (p, q) to $A(\theta_0, \theta_1)$ is a re-expression of the restriction that each θ_j by definition must lie between $\min\{p, 1 - q\}$ and $\max\{p, 1 - q\}$. It is easy to verify that the restriction results in (5.24) being bounded, as values of (p, q) summing to one lie outside $A(\theta_0, \theta_1)$.

Thus upon combining the likelihood and prior the joint posterior density from which we wish to sample can be expressed as

$$f(\theta_0, \theta_1, p, q | s_0, s_1) \quad \propto \quad \theta_0^{s_0}(1 - \theta_0)^{n_0 - s_0}\theta_1^{s_1}(1 - \theta_1)^{n_1 - s_1} \times$$
$$\frac{b(p; \alpha_p, \beta_p)b(q; \alpha_q, \beta_q)}{(p+q-1)^2} I_{A(\theta_0,\theta_1)}(p,q). \quad (5.26)$$

There is no obvious way to simulate draws directly from this four-dimensional distribution.

On the other hand, a joint distribution which approximates (5.26) and from which we can sample easily is given by the density

$$g(\theta_0, \theta_1, p, q | y_0, y_1) \quad = \quad b(\theta_0; s_0 + 1, n_0 - s_0 + 1) \times$$
$$b(\theta_1; s_1 + 1, n_1 - s_1 + 1) \times$$
$$\{k(\theta_0, \theta_1)\}^{-1} \times$$
$$b(p; \alpha_p, \beta_p)b(q; \alpha_q, \beta_q)I_{A(\theta_0,\theta_1)}(p,q), \quad (5.27)$$

where

$$k(\theta_0, \theta_1) \quad = \quad \int\int_{A(\theta_0,\theta_1)} b(p; \alpha_p, \beta_p)b(q; \alpha_q, \beta_q)dp\, dq.$$

Thus (5.27) defines a joint distribution for $(\theta_0, \theta_1, p, q)$ under which marginally θ_0 and θ_1 have independent Beta distributions, while conditionally p and q given (θ_0, θ_1) have independent Beta distributions truncated to $A(\theta_0, \theta_1)$. In particular, (5.27) approximates (5.26) in the sense that the (θ_0, θ_1) marginal under (5.26) is the posterior distribution arising from a uniform prior on (θ_0, θ_1), rather than from the intractable prior that results from marginalizing the actual prior on $(\theta_0, \theta_1, p, q)$ given by (5.24).

The simple form of $A(\theta_0, \theta_1)$ as a union of two rectangles in the unit-square implies that one can readily simulate draws from the joint distribution defined by (5.27) by sampling from the marginal $g(\theta_0, \theta_1)$ and then the conditional $g(p, q | \theta_0, \theta_1)$. In particular, the truncation involved in the latter step is readily handled by evaluating the beta inverse distribution function. Similarly, one can readily compute $k(\theta_0, \theta_1)$ using evaluations of the beta distribution function. This implies that the joint density (5.27) is easily evaluated at any given argument.

Now let $\phi = (\theta_0, \theta_1, p, q)$ denote the entire parameter vector. Our MCMC algorithm for obtaining the next ϕ vector $\phi^{(j+1)}$ given the current vector $\phi^{(j)}$ proceeds by sampling a candidate parameter vector ϕ^* from (5.27) without regard for $\phi^{(j)}$. The Metropolis-Hastings scheme dictates that

$$\phi^{(j+1)} = \begin{cases} \phi^* & \text{with probability} \quad \min\left\{w(\phi^*)/w(\phi^{(j)}), 1\right\}, \\ \phi^{(j)} & \text{with probability} \quad 1 - \min\left\{w(\phi^*)/w(\phi^{(j)}), 1\right\}, \end{cases}$$

where $w(\phi) = f(\phi|s_0, s_1)/g(\phi|s_0, s_1)$ is the ratio of the candidate density to the target density. Note that since the candidate parameter vector is sampled from a distribution not depending on the current parameter vector, the only introduction of serial correlation into the MCMC algorithm is via rejections which lead to the same ϕ vector at successive iterations. Typically we expect that (5.27) will approximate (5.26) well, thereby making the probability of rejection small. By generating candidate (θ_0, θ_1) values from an approximate posterior distribution while generating (p, q) from a modified prior distribution with truncation according to the (θ_0, θ_1) values, we reflect the fact that (θ_0, θ_1) are identifiable, whereas (p, q) are not.

5.6.3 Comparing MCMC Algorithms for the AWU Model of Section 5.2

In the context of the AWU Model of Section 5.2 we compare the performance of the Gibbs sampler and the tailored algorithm for three synthetic datasets. The first dataset consists of 25/250 and 40/250 apparent exposures in the two samples. The second and third datasets involve the same proportions of apparent exposure, but successively four times larger sample sizes. That is, the second dataset comprises 100/1000 and 160/1000 apparent exposures, while the third comprises 400/4000 and 640/4000 apparent exposures. Throughout, $Beta(19, 1)$ priors are assigned to both p and q. This reflects a scenario where the investigator believes the exposure assessment to be very good. Indeed, the prior mode is $(p, q) = (1, 1)$, corresponding to an investigator's best guess that the classification is perfect. However, the prior admits uncertainty about this guess by allowing the possibility that one or both of p and q may be slightly less than one.

Figure 5.11 displays the output of 5000 MCMC iterations for the log odds-ratio ψ, for each dataset and each algorithm. In keeping with our general experience, the performance of the Gibbs sampler worsens as the sample sizes increase. At the smallest of the three sample sizes the performance of the two algorithms seems comparable when assessed 'by eye.' At the largest of sample size, however, the Gibbs sampler is mixing very poorly indeed. On the other hand, there is no obvious change in performance of the tailored algorithm across sample size. In fact the observed rejection rate for the Metropolis-Hastings update does not change appreciably across the three datasets, remaining at about 7% in each case. These findings are commensurate with our experience in this model and related models which are also nonidentifiable. In the face of large sample sizes Gibbs sampling can perform very poorly and it may be necessary to consider more specialized algorithms tailored to the nonidentified nature of the posterior distribution at hand.

5.6.4 MCMC Fitting for the DUAL-DEP Model of Section 5.3

The DUAL-DEP model described in Section 5.3 involves eight unknown parameters,

$$\theta = (r_0, r_1, p_1, p_2, q_1, q_2, \delta_0, \delta_1).$$

As is often the case, it is expedient to augment the parameter vector by the true but unobserved values of V for each subject. Then it is trivial to implement Gibbs sampling updates for r_0 and r_1, as these parameters have beta full conditional posterior distributions, akin to the situation for the simpler DUAL-IND model also described in Section 5.3. The full conditional distributions for the other parameters, however, do not have standard forms. In a related model Dendukuri and Joseph (2001) illustrate that updates according to the full conditional distributions can still be implemented. We are concerned, however, that this may not always work well in light of the nonidentifiable model.

As an alternative we consider block updates to (p_1, p_2, δ_1) and (q_1, q_2, δ_0) given the other parameters and the V values in each case. For instance, let $\lambda = (p_1, p_2, \delta_1)$. The way in which λ governs the distribution of $(V_1^*, V_2^* | V = 1)$ is made explicit by reparameterizing from λ to

$$\phi = (p_1 p_2 + \delta_1, p_1(1 - p_2) - \delta_1, (1 - p_1)p_2 - \delta_1).$$

It is easy to verify that the Jacobian of this transformation is simply one, so that the posterior conditional distribution of ϕ given the other parameters and the data has a density of the form

$$f\left(\phi | \phi^C\right) \propto \phi_1^{c_{1,1}} \phi_2^{c_{1,0}} \phi_3^{c_{0,1}} (1 - \phi_1 - \phi_2 - \phi_3)^{c_{0,0}} f_\lambda(\lambda(\phi)),$$

which is the product of a multinomial likelihood function and a complicated prior density. An obvious Metropolis-Hastings update is to generate a candidate ϕ according to

$$\phi^* \sim \text{Dirichlet}(1 + c_{1,1}, 1 + c_{1,0}, 1 + c_{0,1}, 1 + c_{0,0}), \tag{5.28}$$

regardless of the current ϕ value. Note, in particular, that (5.28) would be the posterior conditional distribution if the prior distribution of ϕ were in fact uniform. Following the usual Metropolis-Hastings scheme, the candidate ϕ^* is accepted with probability

$$acc(\phi^*; \phi) = \min\left\{\frac{f_\lambda(\lambda(\phi^*))}{f_\lambda(\lambda(\phi))}, 1\right\},$$

which is unlikely to be very small given that only a prior density ratio is involved.

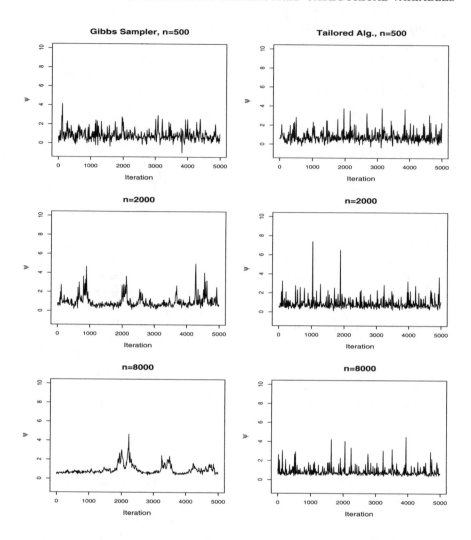

Figure 5.11 *MCMC output for the log odds-ratio ψ under the AWU Model of Section 5.2, using the Gibbs sampler (left panels) and the tailored Metropolis-Hastings algorithm (right panels). The upper panels are based on 25/250 and 40/250 apparent exposures in the control and case samples respectively. The middle and lower panels are based on the same proportions of apparent exposure but respectively four and sixteen times larger sample sizes. In all cases p and q are assigned Beta(19,1) prior distributions.*

5.6.5 Gibbs Sampling for the Model of Section 5.4.3

Applying uniform priors, or more precisely $\theta \sim Dir(1, 1, 1, 1)$, $\phi \sim Dir(1, 1, 1, 1)$, and $r_i \sim Beta(1, 1)$ for $i = 0, 1, 2$, from the multinomial model (5.22) we have

$$f(z, \theta, \phi, r|s) \quad \propto \quad \prod_{i=0}^{2} \prod_{j=1}^{4} \{r_i \theta_j\}^{z_j^{(i)}} \{(1 - r_i)\phi_j\}^{s_j^{(i)} - z_j^{(i)}}.$$

From here we can 'read off' that

$$Z_j^{(i)} | Z_j^{(i) \, C} \quad \sim \quad \text{Binomial}\left(s_j^{(i)}, \frac{r_i \theta_j}{r_i \theta_j + (1 - r_i)\phi_j}\right),$$

$$\theta | \theta^C \quad \sim \quad \text{Dirichlet}\left(1 + \sum_i z_1^{(i)}, \ldots, 1 + \sum_i z_4^{(i)}\right)$$

truncated to the region $\{\theta_1 > \phi_1, \theta_4 < \phi_4\}$,

$$\phi | \phi^C \quad \sim \quad \text{Dirichlet}\left(1 + \sum_i s_1^{(i)} - z_1^{(i)}, \ldots, 1 + \sum_i s_4^{(i)} - z_4^{(i)}\right)$$

truncated to the region $\{\phi_1 < \theta_1, \phi_4 > \theta_4\}$, and finally,

$$r_i | r_i^C \quad \sim \quad \text{Beta}\left(1 + \sum_{j=1}^{4} z_j^{(i)}, 1 + \sum_{j=1}^{4} s_j^{(i)} z_j^{(i)}\right).$$

Thus the Gibbs sampler can be implemented in a straightforward manner.

CHAPTER 6

Further Topics

This chapter discusses some more specialized issues in understanding and adjusting for mismeasurement of explanatory variables. Section 6.1 focusses on a link between measurement error for a continuous variable and misclassification for a binary variable, thereby connecting two previously separate threads in this book. Section 6.2 builds on 6.1 in a particular direction, focussing particularly on the interplay between bias due to mismeasurement and bias due to model misspecification. And finally 6.3 takes a closer look at the issue of model identifiability in Bayesian analysis, particularly as it relates to many mismeasured variable situations.

6.1 Dichotomization of Mismeasured Continuous Variables

Of course one primary feature of this book is its coverage of both mismeasured continuous variables (Chapters 2 and 4) and mismeasured categorical variables (Chapters 3 and 5). To this point only informal contrasts between the two scenarios have been considered. In Chapter 3, for instance, we compared $\alpha \times 100\%$ binary misclassification, in the sense of sensitivity and specificity equal to $1 - \alpha$, to $\alpha \times 100\%$ continuous measurement error, in the sense of $SD(X^*|X) = \alpha SD(X)$. In particular, it was noted that the former can induce much more bias than the latter. Now we turn attention to more formal connections and comparisons, particularly in scenarios where a mismeasured binary variable is in fact *created* from a mismeasured continuous variable.

The present framework involves a binary variable V which is linked to a continuous variable X via thresholding. That is,

$$V = I\{X > c\}, \tag{6.1}$$

for some threshold c. Of course inability to measure X precisely implies inability to measure V precisely. Say X^* is a noisy surrogate for X. Then V^*, a noisy surrogate for V, is defined as

$$V^* = I\{X^* > c\}. \tag{6.2}$$

For instance, say X is serum cholesterol concentration, and physicians regard c as the threshold defining an 'elevated' cholesterol level. Conceptually then it may be of interest to use V rather than X as an explanatory variable in an outcome model. However, if the lab procedure for measuring X actually yields a surrogate X^*, then V^* will be recorded in lieu of V.

To give some idea of how much misclassification is induced by a given amount of measurement error via (6.2), say that X has a normal distribution, taken as $X \sim N(0,1)$ without loss of generality. Moreover, say the surrogate X^* arises via $X^*|X \sim N(X,\tau^2)$. Upon expressing $X^* = X - \tau W$ where (X,W) are independent standard normals, the sensitivity of V^* as a surrogate for V can be expressed as

$$
\begin{aligned}
SN &= Pr(X^* > c|X > c) \\
&= \frac{1}{2} + \{1 - \Phi(c)\}^{-1} \int_0^\infty \{1 - \Phi(c + \tau w)\}\phi(w)\, dw. \qquad (6.3)
\end{aligned}
$$

Here, and throughout this chapter, $\phi()$ and $\Phi()$ denote the standard normal density function and distribution function respectively. The integral in (6.3) must be evaluated numerically. The specificity is determined similarly as

$$
\begin{aligned}
SP &= Pr(X^* < c|X < c) \\
&= \frac{1}{2} + \{\Phi(c)\}^{-1} \int_0^\infty \{\Phi(c - \tau w)\}\phi(w)\, dw. \qquad (6.4)
\end{aligned}
$$

Figure 6.1 conveys the relationship between the magnitude of measurement error in X and the magnitude of misclassification in V. For fixed values of τ, the corresponding values of (SN, SP) arising for various thresholds c are plotted. Clearly $SN = SP$ when $c = 0$, and one can verify that SN decreases with c while SP increases with c. Note that in the present sense $\alpha \times 100\%$ measurement error corresponds to much less than $\alpha \times 100\%$ misclassification. When $c = 0$ for instance, $\tau = 0.1$, $\tau = 0.25$, and $\tau = 0.5$ correspond to $SN = SP = 0.968$, $SN = SP = 0.922$, and $SN = SP = 0.853$ respectively.

For a given threshold c, (6.3) and (6.4) define a magnitude of misspecification (SN, SP) which matches a given magnitude of measurement error τ. And similarly a matching prevalence for V is $r = Pr(X > c) = 1 - \Phi(c)$ when $X \sim N(0,1)$. An obvious comparison to make is between the bias induced by nondifferential measurement error of a given magnitude and that induced by nondifferential misclassification of the matching magnitude. Some such comparisons are given in Table 6.1, in the case of a linear outcome model and no additional precisely measured covariates. That is, the attenuation factor (2.1) for a given τ is compared to the attenuation factor (3.3) for the matching (r, SN, SP), for various values of τ and c. In all instances there is more attenuation under binary misclassification than under continuous measurement error, with the difference being extreme when τ is large and the threshold c is in the tail of the X distribution. Even though 10% measurement error corresponds to much less than 10% misclassification, the latter still leads to more bias than the former.

Table 6.2 considers the scenario where an additional precisely measured covariate is present. Specifically it compares the attenuation factor (2.3) for the X coefficient when Y is regressed on (X^*, Z) instead of (X, Z) to the attenuation factor (3.4) for the V coefficient in the matching misclassification scenario. For illustration $\rho = Cor(X, Z) = 0.8$ is chosen to represent a scenario where the measurement error bias is worsened by substantial correlation between the explanatory variables. To completely determine the matching scenario we take the correlation between the binary predictor V and Z to be

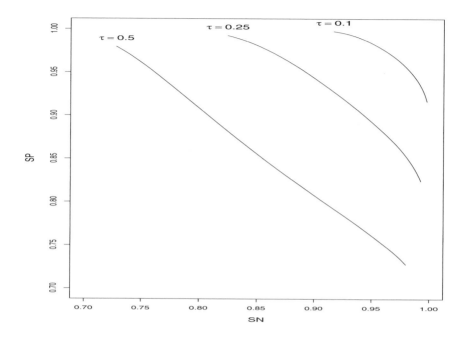

Figure 6.1 *Sensitivity and specificity corresponding to a given magnitude of measurement error under thresholding. For each value of the measurement error standard deviation τ, the plotted values of (SN, SP) correspond to different values of the threshold c, ranging from $c = -2$ to $c = 2$.*

	Meas.	Misclassification		
	Error	$c = 0$	$c = 1$	$c = 2$
$\tau = 0.1$	0.99	0.94	0.93	0.89
$\tau = 0.25$	0.94	0.84	0.81	0.71
$\tau = 0.5$	0.80	0.71	0.63	0.45

Table 6.1 *Attenuation factors under nondifferential measurement error and matching nondifferential misclassification. Different magnitudes of measurement error (τ) and different thresholds (c) are considered.*

$\rho^* = Cor(V, Z) = Cor(I\{X > c\}, Z) = \rho\phi(c)$, assuming now that (X, Z) are jointly normal with standardized marginal distributions. Thus the matching correlation, which is given in the table, depends on the threshold c. Again more attenuation is manifested under misclassification than under measurement error when $\tau = 0.1$ and $\tau = 0.25$, although the situation is reversed when $\tau = 0.5$ and the threshold is not too extreme.

On the face of it Tables 6.1 and 6.2 might be construed as contrasting the impact of mismeasurement before and after dichotomization of the continu-

Misclassification

Meas. Error	$c = 0$ $(\rho^* = 0.32)$	$c = 1$ $(\rho^* = 0.19)$	$c = 2$ $(\rho^* = 0.04)$
$\tau = 0.1$	0.97	0.92	0.92	0.89
$\tau = 0.25$	0.85	0.82	0.80	0.71
$\tau = 0.5$	0.59	0.67	0.61	0.44

Table 6.2 *Attenuation factors under nondifferential measurement error and 'matching' nondifferential misclassification, with an additional precisely measured explanatory variable.*

ous predictor. This is not the case, however. The tables contrast the impact of nondifferential measurement error and nondifferential misclassification in matched scenarios. However, as first pointed out by Flegal, Keyl and Nieto (1991), if a misclassified dichotomous variable is actually created by thresholding a continuous variable subject to nondifferential measurement error, then in general the misclassification will be differential. See also Irwig, Groeneveld and Simpson (1990) and Delpizzo and Borghes (1995) for discussion of misclassification induced by thresholding a mismeasured continuous variable. Initially it seems counter-intuitive that differential misclassification is manifested. If X^* arises from X in a manner which is blind to the outcome variable Y, then $V^* = I\{X^* > c\}$ would also seem to be blind to the value of Y. More generally one might suppose that if X^* is a nondifferential surrogate for X, then $g(X^*)$ would be a nondifferential surrogate for $g(X)$, for any function $g()$. Mathematically, however, conditional independence of X^* and Y given X does not imply conditional independence of $g(X^*)$ and Y given $g(X)$ for an arbitrary function $g()$.

As a more focussed demonstration of the issue, let V and V^* be obtained by thresholding X and X^* at c, as per (6.1) and (6.2), while X^* and Y are conditionally independent given X. We demonstrate that the conditional distribution of V^* given (V, Y) does in fact vary with Y. In particular consider the conditional sensitivity of V^* as a surrogate for V, given $Y = y$. Clearly

$$
\begin{aligned}
Pr(V^* = 1 | V = 1, Y = y) &= Pr(X^* > c | X > c, Y = y) \\
&= E\{Pr(X^* > c | X, Y) | X > c, Y = y\} \\
&= E\{Pr(X^* > c | X) | X > c, Y = y\} \\
&= \int Pr(X^* > c | X = x) f_{X|X>c,Y}(x|y) dx.
\end{aligned}
$$
(6.5)

Of course the probability inside the integral in (6.5) will increase with x, provided X^* is a reasonable surrogate for X. Now say that X and Y are positively associated, i.e., there is some positive relationship between the exposure and the response. Consequently the distribution of $(X | X > c, Y = y)$ will put more mass on larger values of X as y increases, so that (6.5) increases with y. That is, the misclassification is differential.

To give a concrete example say

$$\begin{pmatrix} X \\ Y \end{pmatrix} \sim N\begin{pmatrix} 1 & \omega \\ \omega & 1 \end{pmatrix},$$

while $X^*|X,Y \sim N(X,\tau^2)$. Then the probability inside (6.5) is simply $1 - \Phi\{(c-x)/\tau\}$, while the integration over x is with respect to a $N(\omega y, 1-\omega^2)$ distribution truncated to values larger than c. As a numerical example say $c = 0$ and $\tau = 0.5$, giving an unconditional sensitivity (6.3) of 0.843. Now say that there is substantial dependence between X and Y, with $\omega = 0.5$. Then numerical integration of (6.5) gives the conditional sensitivity as 0.75, 0.79, 0.83, 0.88, and 0.93, for $y = -2, \dots, y = 2$ respectively. Clearly the misclassification is differential to a substantial extent. Moreover, this will be further magnified when the association between X and Y is stronger. For instance when $\omega = 0.9$ the conditional sensitivities range from 0.57 when $y = -2$ to 0.96 when $y = 2$. While the misclassification does arise in a manner which is qualitatively blind to the outcome variable, the end result is a substantial departure from the nondifferential scenario. Following Gustafson and Le (2002) we describe this kind of misclassification as *differential due to dichotomization* (DDD), to distinguish it from the nondifferential situation.

Having established that a mismeasured predictor arising from dichotomization involves differential misclassification, it is clear that the impact of this misclassification may differ from that of nondifferential misclassification as given in Tables 6.1 and 6.2. To investigate this in a simple setting, say that ideally one wishes to fit a linear regression of Y to $V = I\{X > c\}$, but in actuality Y is regressed on $V^* = I\{X^* > c\}$, where X^* is a nondifferential surrogate for X. Clearly

$$E(Y|V^*) \quad = \quad E(Y|V^* = 0) + V^*\{E(Y|V^* = 1) - E(Y|V^* = 0)\},$$

and similarly

$$E(Y|V) \quad = \quad E(Y|V = 0) + V\{E(Y|V = 1) - E(Y|V = 0)\},$$

so the attenuation factor for estimating the V coefficient is simply

$$AF \quad = \quad \frac{E(Y|V^* = 1) - E(Y|V^* = 0)}{E(Y|V = 1) - E(Y|V = 0)}.$$

Upon writing the conditional expectations in iterated fashion, and noting that $E(Y|X, V^*)$ does not depend on V^* since X^* is nondifferential, we have

$$AF \quad = \quad \frac{E\{m(X)|X^* > c\} - E\{m(X)|X^* < c\}}{E\{m(X)|X > c\} - E\{m(X)|X < c\}}, \tag{6.6}$$

where

$$m(x) \quad = \quad E(Y|X = x)$$

is the actual regression function. A first comment about (6.6) is simply that it does depend on the actual distribution of Y given X, via $m(X)$. In contrast, it was stressed in Chapters 2 and 3 that the bias due to nondifferential mismeasurement does not depend on the actual response distribution. Moreover, we know that the bias due to nondifferential measurement error depends on the distribution of X only through the variance of X. In contrast, it is evident that (6.6) depends on the distribution of X in a more detailed manner. Thus claims about the impact of DDD misclassification are likely to be less general than claims about nondifferential mismeasurement.

To consider a special case of (6.6), say that X is normally distributed, assuming without loss of generality that $X \sim N(0,1)$. Also assume that $X^*|X,Y \sim N(X,\tau^2)$, and that $m(X) = \beta_0 + \beta_1 X$, i.e., a linear response model holds. It is clear from the form of (6.6) that $\beta_0 = 0$ and $\beta_1 = 1$ can be assumed without loss of generality. Then the assumed joint normality of (X, X^*) leads easily to

$$AF = \frac{\lambda R(c)}{R(\lambda c)}, \tag{6.7}$$

where $\lambda = (1+\tau^2)^{-1/2}$ and

$$R(z) = \frac{\Phi(z)\{1 - \Phi(z)\}}{\phi(z)},$$

where again $\phi()$ and $\Phi()$ denote the standard normal density function and distribution function respectively. Since $R(z)$ is symmetric and decreasing in $|z|$, it follows that the multiplicative bias (6.7) is a decreasing function of τ, as expected. Also, (6.7) is a decreasing function of $|c|$, so that the bias worsens as the threshold used for dichotomization moves away from the centre of the X distribution.

An obvious question is whether dichotomization makes the impact of mismeasurement better or worse. That is, how does the attenuation factor (6.7) compare to the attenuation factor when Y is regressed on X^* in lieu of X. A particularly clear comparison results when $c = 0$, i.e., the threshold is at the centre of the X distribution. Then the DDD attenuation factor (6.7) is simply $(1+\tau^2)^{-1/2}$, as opposed to $(1+\tau^2)^{-1}$ for nondifferential measurement error. That is, changing the explanatory variable from X to $V = I\{X > 0\}$ involves a *reduction* in bias due to mismeasurement. This is surprising given that generally nondifferential misclassification of a binary variable tends to yield *more* bias than nondifferential measurement error in a continuous variable, as witnessed by Tables 6.1 and 6.2. As a specific example, say $\tau = 0.5$ and $c = 0$. Then the DDD attenuation factor is 0.894 compared to the nondifferential measurement error attenuation factor of 0.8. On the other hand, Table 6.2 gives the nondifferential misclassification attenuation factor as 0.63.

Of course the comparisons above pertain to a threshold $c = 0$ in the centre of the X distribution. As already noted, the DDD attenuation is worse when the threshold is further from the centre of the distribution. It is interesting to note, however, that $R(z) \sim 1/|z|$ as $|z| \to \infty$, so that the attenuation factor (6.7) tends to $(1 + \tau^2)^{-1}$ as $|c|$ tends to infinity. Even in the worst-case of a threshold in the extreme tail of the X distribution, the attenuation due to DDD misclassification is only as bad as the attenuation due to continuous measurement error.

The determination of the DDD attenuation factor is readily extended to situations involving an additional precisely measured explanatory variable. Gustafson and Le (2002) give an expression for the attenuation factor when a linear regression of Y on $(1, V^*, Z)$ is used in lieu of $(1, V, Z)$. In the special case that the actual response relationship is linear, i.e., $E(Y|X, Z)$ is linear in (X, Z), and (X^*, X, Z) have a multivariate normal distribution, this expression specializes to

$$ AF = \lambda \left\{ \frac{R(c) - \rho^2 \phi(c)}{R(\lambda c) - \rho^2 \lambda \phi(\lambda c)} \right\}, \tag{6.8} $$

which clearly reduces to (6.7) when $\rho = Cor(X, Z) = 0$. Gustafson and Le demonstrate that the previously elucidated relationship still holds in this situation, namely (6.8) corresponds to less bias than nondifferential measurement error, which in turn corresponds to less bias than nondifferential misclassification. In addition, they demonstrate similar behaviour in logistic regression scenarios, using numerical techniques akin to those in Chapters 2 and 3.

Gustafson and Le also point out several curious features about the behaviour of (6.8). In particular, for some fixed values of c (6.8) is not monotonically decreasing in $|\rho|$, and for some fixed values of ρ (6.8) is not monotonically decreasing in $|c|$. Thus the impact of DDD misclassification is less generally predictable than that of nondifferential mismeasurement. Some insight into the behaviour is gleaned by noting that for any fixed ρ (6.7) tends to λ^2 as $|c|$ tends to infinity, matching the attenuation due to nondifferential measurement error in the special case that $\rho = 0$. In some sense then an extreme threshold diminishes the impact of correlation between predictors on the mismeasurement bias.

Of course (6.7) and (6.8) describe the attenuation arising in quite narrow settings, with a linear regression function being assumed in particular. In fact the dependence of the attenuation factor on the actual regression function relates to reasons why an analyst might choose to dichotomize a predictor variable in the first place. One may dichotomize to avoid postulating a particular form for the regression relationship. Whereas $E(Y|X)$ may or may not be linear in X, $E(Y|V)$ is necessarily linear in V, since V is binary. On the other hand, of course, information is lost by analyzing (Y, V) rather than (Y, X). Also, dichotomization does not necessarily lead to a correct model in the presence of additional covariates. Nonetheless, dichotomization of predictors is relatively common in statistical practice, even when one can reasonably assume that Y varies with X in a 'smooth' manner. On the other hand, sometimes predictors are dichotomized because it is plausible to posit a threshold regression effect rather than a smooth effect. That is, one may think that $E(Y|X)$ being linear in $V = I\{X > c\}$ is more plausible *a priori* than $E(Y|X)$ being linear in X.

To investigate how the DDD attenuation depends on the actual regression function more thoroughly, say the real regression relationship is

$$m(X) \;\; = \;\; (1 - \omega)X + \omega I\{X > c\},$$

involving a combination of a linear effect and a threshold effect. This is a special case of a scenario investigated by Gustafson and Le (2002) involving an additional precisely measured covariate. The DDD attenuation factor (6.6) is then readily computed as

$$AF \;\; = \;\; \frac{(1 - \omega)a_1 + \omega a_3}{(1 - \omega)a_2 + \omega}, \tag{6.9}$$

where

$$a_1 \;\; = \;\; E(X|X^* > c) - E(X|X^* < c),$$

$$a_2 \;\; = \;\; E(X|X > c) - E(X|X < c),$$

and

$$a_3 \;\; = \;\; 1 - Pr(V = 0|V^* = 1) - Pr(V = 1|V^* = 0).$$

Of course (6.9) reduces to (6.7) when $\omega = 0$, as must be the case. As ω increases to one, however, the attenuation factor increases monotonically to a_3, which is identically the attenuation factor (3.3) in the matching nondifferential misclassification scenario. That is, if $E(Y|X)$ is actually linear in $V = I\{X > c\}$, then the bias matches that incurred by nondifferential misclassification. In fact, under the slightly stronger assumption that the distribution of $Y|X$ depends on X only through $V = I\{X > c\}$, one can verify that $V^* = I\{X^* > c\}$ is actually a nondifferential surrogate for V. Put another way, the extent to which thresholding yields differential misclassification depends strongly on how the conditional distribution of $Y|X$ depends on X. The simple scenario above alludes to a tradeoff. In situations where fitting a threshold variable is more appropriate (ω larger), the mismeasurement bias is closer to that incurred under nondifferential misclassification, i.e., larger. The interplay between the appropriateness of the model and the mismeasurement bias is explored more generally in Section 6.2.

In summary, dichotomization of predictors via thresholding is a scenario where misclassification might appear to be nondifferential, but can in fact be substantially differential. This certainly raises flags about 'off-the-cuff' assumptions of nondifferential mismeasurement. Since the DDD misclassification bias is typically quite modest relative to the nondifferential misclassification bias, there is a risk of overcorrecting for misclassification by incorrectly making the nondifferential assumption. The situation is further muddied given our demonstration that the bias due to DDD misclassification can vary considerably with the actual regression relationship between the outcome variable and the underlying continuous explanatory variable.

We close this section by noting that DDD misclassification can arise without explicit construction of a binary variable from a continuous variable. In many questionnaire-based studies, subjects are asked to dichotomize variables implicitly. For instance, a subject might be asked to place his cumulative exposure to an agent into one of several ordered categories. In a rough sense the mental processes leading to the 'noisy' response for such a question must involve thresholding of an 'internal' X^*. Consequently DDD misclassification is not limited to scenarios whereby an investigator explicitly constructs the dichotomous predictor by thresholding the continuous predictor.

6.2 Mismeasurement Bias and Model Misspecification Bias

In the previous section, the bias induced by DDD misclassification was seen to vary with the actual relationship between the outcome variable and the underlying continuous explanatory variable. This touches on the much broader point that most statistical analyses are susceptible to multiple sources of bias. Of course the emphasis in this book is on understanding and reducing the bias resulting from mismeasured variables. It may not always be reasonable, however, to view this in isolation from other potential biases. The previous findings for DDD misclassification motivate more formal consideration of how biases due to mismeasurement and model misspecification might interact with one another in practice.

There seems to be very little consideration of mismeasurement and model misspecification simultaneously, with the notable exceptions of Lagakos (1988) and Begg and Lagakos (1992, 1993) in a hypothesis-testing context. In a linear model setting, Gustafson (2002a) gives a simple framework for considering bias due to mismeasurement and bias due to model misspecification simultaneously. Consider an outcome variable Y and a pool of k possible predictor variables $X = (X_1, \ldots, X_k)'$, with independent (Y, X) realizations for n subjects. Now say that in fact the 'correct' predictor variables are $S = \{S_1(X), \ldots, S_q(X)\}'$, in the sense that

$$E(Y|X) = \nu_1 S_1(X) + \ldots \nu_q S_q(X), \qquad (6.10)$$

for some coefficients $\nu = (\nu_1, \ldots, \nu_q)'$. Thus an ideal analysis involves linear regression of Y on S. Note that this formulation is very general, as q, the number of correct predictors, need not be the same as m, the number of available predictors. Also, a given S_j can depend on the available predictors in an arbitrary manner, and in particular the actual regression function (6.10) might involve interaction terms or nonlinear terms.

To entertain the possibility of fitting a misspecified model, say that $T = \{T_1(X), \ldots, T_p(X)\}'$ are the regressors chosen for analysis. Moreover, let $\beta = (\beta_1, \ldots, \beta_p)'$ be the large-n limiting coefficients from linear regression of Y on T. Thus with enough data the analysis incorrectly indicates the regression function to be

$$\tilde{E}(Y|X) = \beta_1 T_1(X) + \ldots \beta_p T_p(X). \qquad (6.11)$$

In trying to estimate the regression function then, the difference between (6.11) and (6.10) is the large-sample bias incurred because of model misspecification. We choose to summarize the magnitude of this bias by the average squared-error (ASE), defined as

$$ASE_{SPC} = E\left[\{\beta'T(X) - \nu'S(X)\}^2\right].$$
(6.12)

In particular, the average is with respect to the distribution of the available predictors X, with the view that errors in estimating the regression function at common values of X are more damaging than errors at rare values.

Now say that in fact the chosen predictors T cannot all be measured precisely. Rather $T^* = (T_1^*, \ldots, T_p^*)'$ is the observed surrogate for T. Also, let $\beta^* = (\beta_1^*, \ldots, \beta_p^*)'$ be the large-sample limiting coefficients from linear regression of Y on T^*. If the mismeasurement is ignored or undetected, then with enough data the analysis indicates

$$\tilde{E}^*(Y|X) = \beta_1^* T_1(X) + \ldots \beta_p^* T_p(X)$$
(6.13)

to be the true regression function, i.e., the analysis treats the coefficients from regression of Y on T^* as if they are the coefficients from regression of Y on T. The total bias in estimating the regression function is then the difference between (6.13) and (6.10). In keeping with (6.12) we summarize this via

$$ASE_{TOT} = E\left[\{\beta^{*'}T(X) - \nu'S(X)\}^2\right].$$
(6.14)

Similarly, the difference between (6.13) and (6.11) is naturally regarded as the bias attributed to mismeasurement alone. Thus we also define

$$ASE_{MSR} = E\left[\{\beta^{*'}T(X) - \beta'T(X)\}^2\right].$$
(6.15)

To this point, (6.14) summarizes the joint impact of model misspecification and mismeasurement, while (6.12) and (6.15) describe the respective individual impacts. Perhaps somewhat predictably, it is shown in Gustafson (2002a) that an additive relationship exists, i.e.

$$ASE_{TOT} = ASE_{SPC} + ASE_{MSR}.$$
(6.16)

Also, computable expressions for ASE_{SPC} and ASE_{MSR} are given. These follow easily upon noting that both β and β^* are functions of ν, since the limiting coefficients under a misspecified model necessarily depend on the true relationship between Y and X. In particular, standard large-sample theory for misspecified models (e.g., White 1982) gives

$$\beta = \{E(TT')\}^{-1} E(TS')\nu,$$

and similarly

$$\beta^* = \{E(T^*T^{*'})\}^{-1} E(T^*S')\nu.$$

This leads easily to

$$ASE_{SPC} = \nu' A\nu,$$

where

$$A = E(SS') - E(ST')E(TT')^{-1}E(TS').$$

Similarly,

$$ASE_{MSR} = \nu'B\nu,$$

where

$$B = C'E(TT')C,$$

with

$$C = E(TT')^{-1}E(TS') - E(T^*T^{*'})^{-1}E(T^*S').$$

6.2.1 Further Consideration of Dichotomization

We consider an example where the decomposition (6.16) sheds light on the interplay of model misspecification and mismeasurement. In particular, we build upon the discussion of dichotomization in Section 6.1. Assume that the two available predictors (X, Z) follow a bivariate normal distribution, assuming without loss of generality that both X and Z are standardized to have mean zero and variance one. Also, let $\rho = \text{Cor}(X, Z)$. Now say that the analyst is contemplating whether or not to dichotomize the continuous predictor X. That is, he has two choices of regressors in mind, namely $T^{(C)} = (1, X, Z)'$ and $T^{(D)} = (1, I\{X > 0\}, Z)'$. Note that in the latter case the threshold is at the centre of the X distribution. Also, say that X is subject to nondifferential measurement error which is both unbiased and normally distributed, so that the measured regressors are either $T^{*(C)} = (1, X^*, Z)$ or $T^{*(D)} = (1, I\{X^* > 0\}, Z)$, where $X^*|X, Z, Y \sim N(X, \tau^2)$.

Following the example in Section 6.1, it proves fruitful to consider what happens when the true relationship between the response and predictors falls in between the possibilities considered by the analyst. Specifically, say that

$$
\begin{aligned}
E(Y|X, Z) &= \nu^T S \\
&= \nu_1 + \nu_2 \left\{ (1 - \omega)X + \omega\sqrt{2\pi}\left(I\{X > 0\} - \frac{1}{2}\right) \right\} + \\
&\quad \nu_3 Z,
\end{aligned}
\tag{6.17}
$$

for some $\omega \in [0, 1]$. As ω increases then, $T^{(D)}$ becomes a more appropriate choice of regressors while $T^{(C)}$ becomes a less appropriate choice. As an aside, the centering and scaling of the indicator function in (6.17) appears for a technical reason. In particular, for any value of ω it leads to $\beta = \nu$ when considering $T^{(C)}$ as the predictors. Thus ω is more readily interpreted as the weight given to the dichotomous component in (6.17).

With moderate numerical effort the moments needed to determine ASE_{SPC} and ASE_{MSR} can be computed in this scenario. General considerations discussed in Gustafson (2002a) imply that both terms will depend on ν only through ν_2. Roughly speaking, this follows since only the second of the three regressors is misspecified and subject to mismeasurement. The decomposition

(6.16) thus simplifies to $ASE_{SPC} = A_{22}\nu_2^2$ and $ASE_{MSR} = B_{22}\nu_2^2$. In particular, the ratio of either ASE_{SPC} or ASE_{MSR} to ASE_{TOT} does not depend on ν.

Figure 6.2 plots the terms in the decomposition as functions of ω. Both choices of predictors T are considered, as are different values of ρ and τ. The observed behaviour of the model misspecification term ASE_{SPC} is entirely predictable. If the continuous predictor is used then this term increases with ω, as the true regression function moves away from the postulated form. Similarly, ASE_{SPC} decreases with ω when the dichotomous predictor is used. The mismeasurement term behaves differently for the two choices of predictors. With the continuous predictor, ASE_{MSR} does not depend on ω. This extends the notion from Chapter 2 that the bias due to continuous nondifferential measurement error does not depend on the actual distribution of the outcome variable given the response variable. With the dichotomized predictor, however, ASE_{MSR} increases with ω. This quantifies the tradeoff noted in Section 6.1. With DDD misclassification, the mismeasurement bias increases as the model misspecification bias decreases. This phenomenon is particularly acute in the $\tau = 0.75$ scenarios shown in Figure 6.2. Here ASE_{TOT} actually increases with ω for larger values of ω, so that the overall error *increases* as the true relationship moves closer to the postulated model. That is, the gain in improved model fit is more than offset by the increased bias due to mismeasurement. Generally speaking this tradeoff indicates why it is valuable to consider mismeasurement bias in tandem with other biases rather than in isolation.

6.2.2 Other Examples

Two different examples of using the decomposition (6.16) are given in Gustafson (2002a). The first involves a situation where the analysis is missing a regressor. Specifically the analysis uses $T = (1, X, Z)$ as regressors when in fact either $S = (1, X, Z, X^2)$ or $S = (1, X, Z, XZ)$ are the true regressors. Thus the analysis is ignoring either curvature or interaction which is actually present. Moreover, a nondifferential surrogate X^* is measured in lieu of X. Predictably it turns out that ASE_{SPC} increases with the coefficient on the term in S which is omitted from T. It turns out, however, that ASE_{MSR} decreases with the magnitude of this coefficient. That is the damaging impact of more missed curvature or interaction is partly offset by a reduction in bias due to mismeasurement. This constitutes another situation where ASE_{SPC} and ASE_{MSR} are inversely related as the underlying regression relationship changes.

The other example in Gustafson (2002a) involves forming m binary variables from a continuous variable X. That is, the analysis proceeds with

$$T = (I_{A_1}(X), \ldots, I_{A_m}(X), Z)'$$

taken to be the predictors, where the disjoint intervals $(A_1, \ldots A_m)$ partition the real line. Because of measurement error, however, the recorded predictors

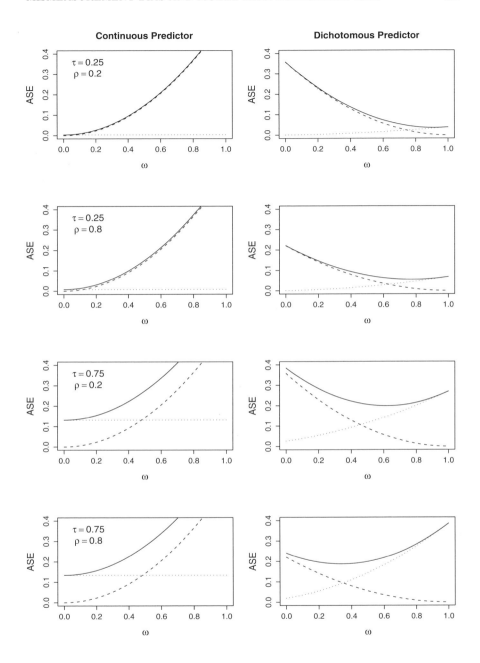

Figure 6.2 ASE_{TOT} (solid curve), ASE_{SPC} (dashed curve), and ASE_{MSR} (dotted curve) as a function of ω which indexes the true relationship (6.17). The four pairs of plots correspond to combinations of $\tau = 0.25$ or $\tau = 0.75$ and $\rho = 0.2$ or $\rho = 0.8$. For each pair, the left plot corresponds to $T^{(C)} = (1, X, Z)'$ as the postulated predictors, while the right plot corresponds to $T^{(D)} = (1, I\{X > 0\}, Z)'$ as the postulated predictors. The vertical scaling of the plots is based on $\nu_2 = 1$.

are

$$T^* = (I_{A_1}(X^*), \ldots, I_{A_m}(X^*), Z)',$$

where X^* is an unbiased and nondifferential surrogate for X. The true regression function is taken to be simply linear, i.e., $S = (1, X, Z)$. With lots of data one can argue for selecting a large number m of indicator functions, to better approximate the unknown shape of the actual regression function. Indeed, ASE_{SPC} decreases with m. This is partially offset, however, by ASE_{MSR} which increases with m. Once again the two biases are inversely related. It almost seems as if a 'no-free-lunch' principle is at play, as steps taken to reduce the impact of model misspecification may well lead to increased error due to mismeasurement, and vice versa.

Another aspect of the interplay between model misspecification and mismeasurement emphasized in Gustafson (2002a) is that mismeasurement impairs the ability of standard diagnostic procedures to detect model misspecification. In situations where clear model violations would be evident from residual plots based on (Y, X), the analogous plots based on (Y, X^*) may appear to be in order. This can arise simply because the noise associated by observing X^* rather than X blurs the pattern in the plot. Hence it seems reasonable to develop flexible Bayesian response models for mismeasurement adjustment. Indeed, flexible response models may prove to have greater utility than flexible exposure models. This topic has not received much attention in the literature, and is ripe for further research. Berry, Carroll and Ruppert (2002) and Mallick, Hoffman and Carroll (2002) are recent papers with interesting work in this direction.

6.3 Identifiability in Mismeasurement Models

Consider a statistical model for observable data y given a parameter vector θ, expressed via a density function $f(y|\theta)$. The model is said to be *identifiable* if $f(y|\theta_1) = f(y|\theta_2)$ for all y implies that $\theta_1 = \theta_2$. Intuitively, a *nonidentifiable* model lacking this property cannot yield consistent estimators of θ as a whole. In particular say θ_1 and θ_2 are distinct values of θ violating the property above, and say that in fact θ_1 is the true parameter vector. Clearly data alone cannot shed light on whether θ_1 is a more plausible parameter value than θ_2, even with a very large sample size.

Often issues of parameter identifiability are quite central to models which account for mismeasurement, since a great deal must be known about the mismeasurement process in order to obtain a fully identified model. This is particularly true in scenarios where neither gold-standard measurements or pure replicate measurements can be obtained. We have already alluded to problems of nonidentifiability in Chapter 5. For instance, the model in Section 5.2 involving partial knowledge of misclassification probabilities is formally nonidentifiable, though the findings there suggest that reasonably good partial knowledge can still lead to useful inferences. In this section we take a closer look at the utility of mismeasurement models that lack formal parameter identifiability.

6.3.1 Estimator Performance in Nonidentified Models

We start with a general discussion of how much can be learned about a parameter of interest from a Bayes analysis with a nonidentifiable model. The general treatment follows Gustafson (2002b), which in turn builds on early investigations in specific nonidentifiable models (Neath and Samaniego 1997; Gustafson, Le and Saskin 2001). Say the model in question is initially parameterized by a vector θ with p components. This can be thought of as the 'obvious' parameterization for scientific purposes, and the parameterization under which the prior distribution is specified in particular. Thus a model density $f(\text{data}|\theta)$ and a prior density $f(\theta)$ are at hand.

To gain insight regarding identifiability, we seek to reparameterize from the original parameter vector θ to $\phi = (\phi_I, \phi_N)$, in such a way that $f(\text{data}|\phi) = f(\text{data}|\phi_I)$. That is, the distribution of the data depends only on ϕ_I, which we call the identifiable component of ϕ, and not on ϕ_N, the nonidentifiable component. We call such a parameterization *transparent*, as it is intended to make apparent the impact of nonidentifiability. Of course the prior distribution $f(\theta)$ as specified in the original parameterization can be transformed to $f(\phi)$ in the transparent parameterization. Indeed, along the lines of Dawid (1979), it is useful to think of the prior for ϕ in terms of the marginal density $f(\phi_I)$ and the conditional density $f(\phi_N|\phi_I)$. Then immediately Bayes theorem gives

$$f(\phi_I|\text{data}) \quad \propto \quad f(\text{data}|\phi_I)f(\phi_I), \qquad (6.18)$$

while

$$f(\phi_N|\phi_I, \text{data}) \quad = \quad f(\phi_N|\phi_I). \qquad (6.19)$$

Thus (6.18), the posterior marginal distribution for ϕ_I, is typically governed by the regular asymptotic theory that applies to identifiable models. In particular, the posterior marginal distribution of ϕ_I converges to a point mass at the true value of ϕ_I as the sample size increases. Alternately, (6.19), the posterior conditional distribution for $\phi_N|\phi_I$, is identical to the prior conditional distribution. There is no Bayesian learning whatsoever about this conditional distribution.

Often a simple and reasonable choice of prior for θ will involve independent components, i.e., $f(\theta) = f(\theta_1)\ldots f(\theta_p)$. However, the induced prior $f(\phi)$ may involve substantial dependence between components, and dependence between ϕ_I and ϕ_N specifically. This has implications, as the posterior marginal density for ϕ_N is

$$f(\phi_N|\text{data}) \quad = \quad \int f(\phi_N|\phi_I)f(\phi_I|\text{data})d\phi_I,$$

which does not in general reduce to the prior marginal $f(\phi_N)$, unless ϕ_I and ϕ_N are *a priori* independent. Whereas conditionally there is no learning or updating about ϕ_N given ϕ_I, marginally there can be some learning about ϕ_N from the data. We refer to this as *indirect learning*, as it is learning about ϕ_N that results only because of, or via, learning about ϕ_I.

Now consider a scalar parameter of interest ψ, which, while initially defined in terms of the θ parameterization, can be expressed as a function of ϕ equally well. Thus we write $\psi = g(\phi)$. We can estimate ψ by its posterior mean, given as

$$
\begin{aligned}
E(\psi|\text{data}) &= E\{g(\phi_I, \phi_N)|\text{data}\} \\
&= \int \int g(\phi_I, \phi_N) f(\phi_I, \phi_N|\text{data}) \, d\phi_N \, d\phi_I \\
&= \int \int g(\phi_I, \phi_N) f(\phi_N|\phi_I) \, d\phi_N \, f(\phi_I|\text{data}) \, d\phi_I \\
&= E\{\tilde{g}(\phi_I)|\text{data}\},
\end{aligned}
$$

where

$$
\tilde{g}(\phi_I) = \int g(\phi_I, \phi_N) f(\phi_N|\phi_I) d\phi_N.
$$

Thus the posterior mean of $\psi = g(\phi_I, \phi_N)$ is identically the posterior mean of $\tilde{g}(\phi_I)$, which of course is a function of the identifiable parameter component alone.

Given the re-expression of the posterior mean in terms of ϕ_I alone, under weak regularity conditions the large-sample behaviour of the estimator $E(\psi|\text{data})$ is described by the usual asymptotic theory applied to the identifiable model $f(\text{data}|\phi_I)$. That is, if the model is correct and a sample of size n yields $\hat{\psi}^{(n)} = E(\psi|\text{data})$, then

$$
n^{1/2}\left\{\hat{\psi}^{(n)} - \tilde{g}(\phi_I)\right\} \Rightarrow N\left[0, \{\tilde{g}'(\phi_I)\}' I(\phi_I)^{-1}\{\tilde{g}'(\phi_I)\}\right]
$$

in distribution, as $n \to \infty$. Here $I(\phi_I)$ is the Fisher information matrix based on $f(\text{data}|\phi_I)$ for a single datapoint. Of course the estimator is biased, as it converges to $\tilde{g}(\phi_I)$ rather than $g(\phi_I, \phi_N)$ as desired. Indeed, considering both bias and variance, the mean-squared-error (MSE) incurred when estimating ψ by $\hat{\psi}^{(n)}$ can be approximated as

$$
\begin{aligned}
MSE \approx\ &\{\tilde{g}(\phi_I) - g(\phi_I, \phi_N)\}^2 + \\
&n^{-1}\{\tilde{g}'(\phi_I)\}' I(\phi_I)^{-1}\{\tilde{g}'(\phi_I)\}, \quad\quad\quad (6.20)
\end{aligned}
$$

where the first term is the squared asymptotic bias and the second term is large-sample approximate variance. Despite being very easy to establish, this approach to quantifying the frequentist performance of a posterior mean in a nonidentified model does not seem to have been pursued prior to Gustafson (2002b).

Given a prior and true value for θ, (6.20) indicates how well a parameter of interest can be estimated. Thus we can investigate how much prior information is needed to overcome the lack of identifiability and obtain useful inferences. In many mismeasurement models ϕ_N will be of dimension one or two, making it feasible to compute $\tilde{g}()$ and its derivatives numerically if no closed-form exists. While indirect learning is discussed less formally in the next example, the subsequent example of Section 6.3.3 uses (6.20) explicitly.

6.3.2 Example: Partial Knowledge of Misclassification Probabilities Revisited

We return to the scenario of Section 5.2, to examine the impact of nonidentifiability more closely when only partial information about misclassification probabilities is available. Recall that the goal is to make inferences about the odds-ratio in a case-control scenario with nondifferential misclassification of the binary exposure. The initial parameterization is $\theta = (r_0, r_1, p, q)$, where r_i is the exposure prevalence in the i-th population ($i = 0$ corresponding to controls, $i = 1$ corresponding to cases), while (p, q) are the sensitivity and specificity of exposure misclassification. As alluded to in Section 5.2, a transparent parameterization involves $\phi_I = (\theta_0, \theta_1)$ and $\phi_N = (p, q)$, where θ_i is the prevalence of apparent exposure in the i-th population.

Say the investigator starts with an independence prior in the original parameterization, assigning uniform priors to the prevalences r_0 and r_1, and priors with densities $f(p)$ and $f(q)$ to p and q respectively. Then a slight extension of the developments in Section 5.6.2 gives the conditional prior density of ϕ_N given ϕ_I as

$$f(p, q|\theta_0, \theta_1) \propto \frac{1}{(p + q - 1)^2} f(p) f(q) I_{A(\theta_0, \theta_1)}(p, q), \qquad (6.21)$$

where $A(\theta_0, \theta_1)$ is the union of two rectangles in the unit square, as defined in (5.25). In particular, A consists of (p, q) values which are componentwise greater than $(p, q) = (\max\{\theta_0, \theta_1\}, 1 - \min\{\theta_0, \theta_1\})$, and values which are componentwise less than $(p, q) = (\min\{\theta_0, \theta_1\}, 1 - \max\{\theta_0, \theta_1\})$. Note also that the $(p + q - 1)^{-2}$ term in (6.21) arises from the Jacobian associated with reparameterization.

Bearing in mind that as the sample size grows the posterior distribution on (p, q) will converge to (6.21) evaluated at the true values of (θ_0, θ_1), we see that indirect learning is manifested in two ways. First, the shape of the density on (p, q) is modified by the multiplicative term $(p + q - 1)^{-2}$. On first glance one might think this to have great impact, as this term tends to infinity along the $q = 1 - p$ line in the unit square. However, this line necessarily lies entirely outside the support set $A(\theta_0, \theta_1)$, thereby limiting the influence of this term. Second, the support set may exclude regions with substantial probability under the marginal prior $f(p)f(q)$, thereby making the conditional prior (6.21) more concentrated than the marginal prior.

As a specific example, say the investigator selects identical Beta priors for p and q, both with mean 0.8 and standard deviation 0.075. In particular this yields the $Beta(21.96, 5.49)$ distribution. Again this sort of prior might be viewed as a quantification of quite crude knowledge that the exposure assessments are good but not perfect. A (p, q) scatterplot of a simulated sample from this prior is given in the upper-left panel of Figure 6.3. Now say that in

scenario	r_0	r_1	θ_0	θ_1
(i)	0.0625	0.9375	0.15	0.85
(ii)	0.375	0.625	0.4	0.6
(iii)	0.0625	0.1250	0.15	0.2

Table 6.3 *Three scenarios for prevalence of actual and apparent exposure in a case-control study. The prevalences of apparent exposure (θ_0, θ_1) are obtained from the prevalences of actual exposure (r_0, r_1) via nondifferential misclassification with sensitivity $p = 0.9$ and specificity $q = 0.9$.*

fact the true values of both p and q are 0.9, i.e., each is slightly more than one prior SD away from the prior mean. This typifies a situation where the prior distribution is neither spectacularly good or bad as a representation of the actual truth. Finally, consider three possible values of the exposure prevalences (r_0, r_1). These are given along with the implied apparent exposure prevalences (θ_0, θ_1) in Table 6.3. Note in particular that scenario (iii) might be quite realistic for case-control studies.

For prevalences (i) the upper-right panel of Figure 6.3 displays a sample from the limiting posterior marginal distribution of (p, q), i.e., the prior conditional distribution (6.21) evaluated at the true values of (θ_0, θ_1). Note that truncation has a very considerable and desirable impact, forcing the limiting posterior distribution to be very concentrated near the true values of (p, q) relative to the prior distribution. Thus considerable learning about (p, q) can occur. For prevalences (ii), however, the impact of truncation is almost negligible (lower-left panel of Figure 6.3). In this instance the multiplicative effect of the $(p + q - 1)^{-2}$ term is apparent from the plot, though the discrepancy between the prior and limiting posterior distributions is quite mild. Thus little can be learned about (p, q) from the data in this scenario. Finally, prevalences (iii) lead to considerable learning about the specificity q but virtually no learning about the sensitivity p (lower-right panel of Figure 6.3).

The overall message from Figure 6.3 is that the the efficacy of indirect learning about $\phi_N = (p, q)$ is quite unpredictable. For a given prior distribution and true value for ϕ_N, the amount of indirect learning varies dramatically with the true value of ϕ_I, from very considerable with prevalences (i), to very slight with prevalences (ii). We find this sort of unpredictability to be the norm with nonidentified mismeasurement models. In essence it seems desirable to formulate the best prior possible to permit the *possibility* of benefiting from indirect learning, but in advance one cannot count on such learning taking place to a substantial extent.

In the present inferential scenario, Gustafson, Le and Saskin (2001) compare using a prior on (p, q) to treating (p, q) as known. More precisely they consider 'best guess' values for (p, q), and compare the posterior distribution arising from a prior distribution centred at the guessed values to the posterior distribution arising from pretending that the guessed values are known true values. The latter approach gains identifiability at the cost of model misspecification.

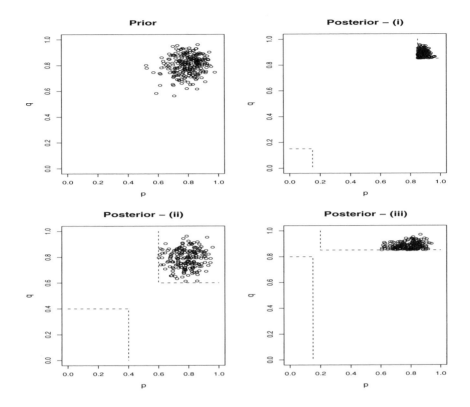

Figure 6.3 *Prior and limiting posterior distributions for* (p, q)*. Each panel gives* (p, q) *scatterplots of a sample from the distribution in question. The upper-left panel gives the prior distribution, while the remaining panels give the large-sample limiting posterior distributions under prevalences (i), (ii), and (iii) as described in the text. The true values are* $(p, q) = (0.9, 0.9)$ *throughout. The dashed lines delineate the rectangles* $A(\theta_0, \theta_1)$*comprising the support of the limiting posterior distribution.*

Of course there is a generic argument in favour of assigning prior distributions to quantities which are genuinely unknown, to more fully account for all the uncertainties at play. In the present setting then, one might expect that admitting uncertainty about (p, q) would result in wider posterior distributions for parameters of interest. Indeed, for some underlying parameter values Gustafson, Le and Saskin (2001) find this to be the case. That is, credible intervals arising from a prior on (p, q) are wider on average, but have higher empirical coverage probabilities than those arising from fixed (p, q). For other underlying parameter values, however, using a prior gives credible intervals that are *both* shorter on average and have higher empirical coverage than their fixed (p, q) counterparts. In particular, this occurs when substantial indirect learning occurs. Surprisingly, even though the data do not inform us directly about ϕ_N, there are circumstances where admitting uncertainty about ϕ_N a *priori* can actually lead to decreased uncertainty about parameters of interest *a posteriori*!

6.3.3 Linear and Normal Models Revisited

Here we revisit the combination of linear and normal measurement, outcome, and exposure models, as discussed in Chapter 4. In particular, say the regression of Y on X is of interest, but only (X^*, Y) can be observed, where X^* is a surrogate for X. The measurement, outcome, and exposure models are taken to be

$$
\begin{aligned}
X^*|X,Y &\sim N(X, \gamma\lambda^2), \\
Y|X &\sim N(\beta_0 + \beta_1 X, \sigma^2), \\
X &\sim N(\alpha_0, \lambda^2).
\end{aligned}
$$

Note that the parameter γ is used to describe the ratio of $Var(X^*|X)$ to $Var(X)$, i.e., γ is interpretable as the measurement error magnitude expressed in relative terms. Note also that this parameterization is particularly relevant in the common scenario that X and X^* are logarithmic transformations of positive variables thought to be related via a multiplicative measurement error relationship.

It is easy to verify that if all six parameters $\theta = (\beta_0, \beta_1, \alpha_0, \sigma^2, \lambda^2, \gamma)$ are unknown then the model is nonidentifiable. Essentially the model assumes that (X^*, Y) have a bivariate normal distribution, so that at most five parameters can be estimated consistently. Toward applying the ideas of Section 6.3.1, note that a transparent parameterization obtains by taking $\phi_I = (\tilde{\beta}_0, \tilde{\beta}_1, \tilde{\alpha}_0, \tilde{\lambda}^2, \tilde{\sigma}^2)$ and $\phi_N = \gamma$, where

$$
\begin{aligned}
\tilde{\beta}_0 &= \beta_0 + \alpha_0 \beta_1/(1+\gamma), \\
\tilde{\beta}_1 &= \beta_1/(1+\gamma), \\
\tilde{\alpha}_0 &= \alpha_0, \\
\tilde{\sigma}^2 &= \sigma^2 + \beta_1^2 \lambda^2 \gamma/(1+\gamma), \\
\tilde{\lambda}^2 &= \lambda^2(1+\gamma),
\end{aligned}
$$

so that

$$
\begin{aligned}
Y|X^* &\sim N(\tilde{\beta}_0 + \tilde{\beta}_1 X^*, \tilde{\sigma}^2), \\
X^* &\sim N(\tilde{\alpha}_0, \tilde{\lambda}^2).
\end{aligned}
$$

Now say a prior of the form

$$
f(\beta_0, \beta_1, \alpha_0, \sigma^2, \lambda^2, \gamma) = f_1(\beta_0) f_2(\beta_1) f_3(\alpha_0) f_4(\sigma^2) f_5(\lambda^2) f_6(\gamma)
$$

is assigned in the original parameterization. One can verify that the $\theta \to \phi$ reparameterization has unit Jacobian, and consequently the conditional prior for $\phi_N|\phi_I$ takes the form

$$
f(\gamma|\beta_0^*, \beta_1^*, \mu_*, \sigma_*^2, \lambda_*^2) \propto f_2\left(\tilde{\beta}_1(1+\gamma)\right) \times
$$

$$f_4\left(\tilde{\sigma}^2 - \gamma\tilde{\beta}_1^2\tilde{\lambda}^2\right) \times$$

$$f_5\left(\tilde{\lambda}^2/(1+\gamma)\right) \times$$

$$f_6(\gamma)I_{\left(0,m(\tilde{\beta}_1,\tilde{\sigma}^2,\tilde{\lambda}^2)\right)}(\gamma), \qquad (6.22)$$

where

$$m\left(\tilde{\beta}_1,\tilde{\sigma}^2,\tilde{\lambda}^2\right) \;=\; \min\left\{\frac{\tilde{\sigma}^2}{\tilde{\beta}_1^2\tilde{\lambda}^2},1\right\}.$$

Thus there is potential for indirect learning here, through both the multiplicative terms which act on $f_6(\gamma)$ in (6.22), and the truncation that arises if $m()$ is less than one.

The nature of indirect learning in this context is investigated by elaborating on an example from Gustafson (2002b). Consider the true parameter values $\gamma = 0.3$, $\beta_0 = 0$, $\alpha_0 = 0$, $\sigma^2 = 0.25$, and $\lambda^2 = 1$. Three different true values for β_1 are considered, namely $\beta_1 = 0.5$, $\beta_1 = 1$, and $\beta_1 = 1.5$. Prior independence in the initial parameterization is assumed, with the priors for β_0, β_1, and α_0 taken to be $N(0,1)$ and the priors for σ^2 and λ^2 taken to be $IG(0.5,0.5)$. Such priors might be appropriate if the data are standardized before analysis. Finally a prior of the form $\gamma \sim Beta(a,b)$ is specified, with four possible values for the hyperparameters considered. In case (i), $(a,b) = (1,1)$, i.e., γ has a uniform prior distribution. In the remaining instances (a,b) are selected to attain a desired prior mean and standard deviation. Specifically prior (ii) is taken to yield $E(\gamma) = 0.4$, $SD(\gamma) = 0.1$, while prior (iii) gives $E(\gamma) = 0.2$, $SD(\gamma) = 0.1$. In both cases the true value of $\gamma = 0.3$ is one prior standard deviation away from the prior mean, again representing priors of 'typical' quality in representing the truth. Prior (iv) is also of typical quality in this sense, with $E(\gamma) = 0.35$, $SD(\gamma) = 0.05$. This smaller prior standard deviation corresponds to sharper prior information than in (ii) or (iii).

For each choice of prior and each true value of β_1, Figure 6.4 plots the conditional density (6.22) evaluated at the true value of ϕ_I. Recall that this is the large-sample limiting posterior marginal distribution for γ, and by comparing this density to the prior density we see how much can be learned about γ from the data. The figure shows that the amount of learning varies greatly across the different priors and across the underlying value of β_1. Generally, when the updating is appreciable it is also desirable. That is, when the data do influence the prior they do 'push' toward the true value of γ. Also, there tends to be more updating when the underlying value of β_1 is larger. In comparing priors (ii) and (iii) we see more ability to push prior (ii) to the left than to push prior (iii) to the right. This is due to the truncation in (6.22), which can eliminate larger values of γ. In comparing priors (ii) and (iv) more updating is seen with the former, presumably because it is a less concentrated prior distribution initially. Overall the findings are in keeping with our general impression in the previous subsection — the extent to which indirect learning occurs is quite unpredictable.

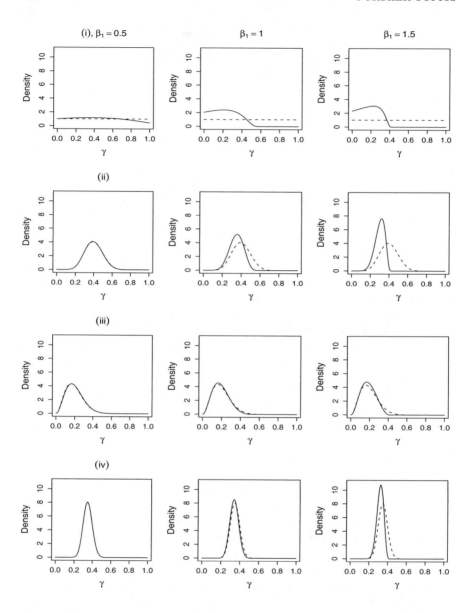

Figure 6.4 *Prior and limiting posterior densities for* γ*. Each panel gives the prior marginal density as a dotted curve and the limiting posterior density (equivalently the prior conditional density) as a solid curve. The rows correspond to Beta priors (i) through (iv) described in the text, while the columns correspond to different underlying values of* β_1*.*

prior	$\beta_1 = 0.5$	$\beta_1 = 1$	$\beta_1 = 1.5$
(i)	0.78	0.39	0.58
(ii)	0.99	0.50	0.01
(iii)	0.97	1.06	1.13
(iv)	1.00	0.83	0.38

Table 6.4 *Ratio of absolute asymptotic bias in using a prior on* γ *versus pretending* γ *is known, when estimating* β_1*. The columns correspond to priors (i) through (iv) as described in the text. The rows correspond to different underlying values of* β_1*. Note that the layout matches that of Figure 6.4*

With some knowledge about γ, one alternative to using a prior distribution is simply to fix γ at a 'best guess' value. This is the notion of 'adjusting with false certainty' first discussed in Section 5.2. While this strategy leads to identifiability, the model will be somewhat misspecified unless the guess is correct. To explore this tradeoff we consider the same scenarios as portrayed in Figure 6.4, with the guessed value of γ matching the prior mean for γ in all instances. For estimating β_1, Table 6.4 gives the ratio of absolute asymptotic bias when using the prior on γ to the absolute asymptotic bias when γ is fixed. Recall from Section 6.3.1 that the bias in the former case is given as $\tilde{g}(\phi_I) - g(\phi_I, \phi_N)$, and note that $\tilde{g}(\phi_I)$ is readily computed via one-dimensional numerical integration with respect to (6.22).

Not surprisingly, Table 6.4 shows a ratio of absolute biases close to one in scenarios where little indirect learning is manifested in Figure 6.4. If the data contain virtually no information about γ, then similar point estimates arise from either using a prior on γ or fixing γ at a commensurate value. On the other hand, scenarios where appreciable indirect learning occurs lead to much less bias when a prior is assigned to γ. That is, the use of a prior allows the data to push toward the true value of γ, which of course cannot happen if γ is fixed in advance. In general then, the use of a reasonable prior may or may not lead to a substantial reduction in bias, but it is very unlikely to produce a substantial increase in bias.

To consider both bias and variance, Table 6.5 gives the approximate $RMSE$ when estimating β_1 with a sample of size $n = 500$ and a prior distribution on γ. This is computed as the square-root of (6.20). Again the different priors on γ and different underlying values of β_1 match those in Figure 6.4. The overall impression is that the $RMSE$ tends to be quite small in absolute terms, to the extent that inferences of useful precision can be drawn even with a uniform prior distribution on γ, or in scenarios where virtually no indirect learning occurs. As a point of comparison, the last row of Table 6.5 gives the $RMSE$ for the naive estimator which doesn't account for mismeasurement, i.e., the slope coefficient from regression of Y on X^*. In all cases these $RMSE$ values are considerably larger than those arising from the mismeasurement model, indicating that the attempted adjustment is well worthwhile even without good prior information on γ. For instance, over the four priors and three

prior	$\beta_1 = 0.5$		$\beta_1 = 1$		$\beta_1 = 1.5$	
	RMSE	(%DTB)	RMSE	(%DTB)	RMSE	(%DTB)
(i)	0.065	(86%)	0.065	(82%)	0.138	(94%)
(ii)	0.048	(62%)	0.049	(61%)	0.039	(0%)
(iii)	0.045	(68%)	0.087	(88%)	0.136	(93%)
(iv)	0.035	(30%)	0.047	(47%)	0.045	(25%)
NAIVE	0.117	(97%)	0.232	(99%)	0.348	(99%)

Table 6.5 *Approximate Root-Mean-Squared-Error (RMSE) in estimating β_1 with a sample size of $n = 500$. The fraction of the mean-squared-error due to bias, i.e., the ratio of squared bias to MSE, is given as the percentage due to bias (%DTB). As previously, the rows and columns correspond to different priors and different underlying values of β_1. The last row corresponds to naive estimation which ignores the measurement error.*

prior	$\beta_1 = 0.5$	$\beta_1 = 1$	$\beta_1 = 1.5$
(i)	0.78	0.41	0.58
(ii)	0.98	0.57	0.31
(iii)	0.97	1.04	1.11
(iv)	1.00	0.88	0.61

Table 6.6 *Ratio of approximate RMSE using a prior on γ to pretending γ is known, when estimating β_1 with a sample size of $n = 500$. The columns correspond to priors (i) through (iv) as described in the text. The rows correspond to different underlying values of β_1. Note that the layout matches that of Figure 6.4.*

values of β_1, the largest ratio of $RMSE$ to β_1 occurs with the uniform prior (i) and $\beta_1 = 0.5$. Even in this worst-case, however, the $RMSE$ is an order of magnitude smaller than that achieved by the naive estimator.

Table 6.5 also reports the percentage of the MSE that is due to squared-bias rather than variance. It is interesting to note that in most cases the bias contribution does not dominate the variance contribution, despite the relatively large sample size. Given this, we revisit the comparisons of Table 6.4 between using a prior on γ and fixing γ at the corresponding best guess. In particular, Table 6.6 reports the ratio of $RMSE$ using a prior to $RMSE$ with γ fixed. Again the table indicates ratios much less than one in instances where substantial indirect learning occurs, and ratios near one otherwise.

6.3.4 Dual Exposure Assessment in One Population

Section 5.3 considered dual assessment of a binary exposure in a case-control setting, and the DUAL-IND model described there is applicable more generally to problems with two misclassified surrogates measured in two populations. In particular, recall that an identifiable six-parameter model results under the strong assumptions that the exposure assessments are nondifferential and conditionally independent of one another given the true exposure.

On the other hand, it is easy to verify that identifiability is lost if the assessments are made in only one population. Notwithstanding this, Joseph, Gyorkos and Coupal (1995) consider dual exposure assesesment in a single population, focussing on Bayesian inference about the exposure prevalence and the four misclassification probabilities. They use a uniform prior on the exposure prevalence, but relatively informative priors on the misclassification probabilities.

Johnson, Gastwirth and Pearson (2001) criticize the approach of Joseph *et al.*, particularly because it lacks identifiability. They argue that one should always split the population under study into two distinct sub-populations or strata, as a route to the identifiable DUAL-IND model. While they are not very prescriptive about how this splitting might be done in practice, demographic variables that are routinely collected in epidemiological investigations could be used for this purpose. For instance, one can imagine using gender or age to define two strata.

On the face of it the argument of Johnson *et al.* seems compelling. Why work with a nonidentifiable model if the data can be augmented easily to yield an identifiable model? As noted in Section 5.3, however, the identifiability breaks down in the special case that both strata have identical exposure prevalences, i.e., $r_0 = r_1$ in the notation used previously. Intuitively, this confirms that identifiability cannot be obtained by flipping coins to split the sampled units into two strata. Further in this vein, it may also be difficult to obtain precise inferences if the prevalences differ only modestly from one another. For instance, unless there is reason to believe that the exposure prevalence varies markedly with gender, stratifying according to gender may be a poor strategy. Perhaps then there are circumstances where it is reasonable to proceed as in Joseph *et al.* with a single population.

To explore this issue, Gustafson (2002b) uses the ideas of 6.3.1 to assess how well the exposure prevalence can be estimated in a single population, using subjective, though not terribly precise, prior distributions on the misclassification probabilities. In this setting the five-dimensional initial parameterization $\theta = (r, p_1, q_1, p_2, q_2)$ involves the exposure prevalence and the four misclassification probabilities for the two assessments. The reparameterization to $\phi = (\phi_I, \phi_N)$ involves taking ϕ_N to be three cell probabilities which determine the joint distribution of the two assessments, while ϕ_N is conveniently taken to be the exposure prevalence r plus any one of the four misclassification probabilities. Two-dimensional integration can then be used to compute $\tilde{g}(\phi_I)$ and its derivatives, as needed to compute the approximate MSE using (6.20).

At least for the particular choices of priors and underlying parameter values investigated in Gustafson (2002b), reasonably precise inferences can result from relatively crude priors. In particular, scenarios where the same Beta prior is assigned to each of p_1, q_1, p_2, q_2 are considered, as representations of a rough belief that the two assessments are 'good but not perfect.' Note in particular that such a prior does not attempt to distinguish between the two assessments, or between the sensitivity and specificity for a given assessment.

The striking finding is that the resulting estimator performance can be better than that achieved by dichotomizing the population and using the DUAL-IND model, even if the sub-population prevalences differ to some extent. In short, consideration of the nonidentifiable model performance leads to a tempering of the recommendation in Johnson *et al.* Splitting the population to achieve identifiability will not always lead to improved estimator performance.

6.4 Further Remarks

The topics discussed in this chapter appear outwardly to be somewhat idiosyncratic. In all cases, though, they relate to broad issues in understanding and correcting for mismeasurement of explanatory variables. And generally speaking, all three topics are ripe for further research. The consideration of DDD misclassification in Section 6.1 points to how differential mismeasurement can arise easily and subtly, and reinforces the notion that differential mismeasurement can have quite a different impact than nondifferential mismeasurement. In Section 6.2 the decomposition of error in estimating a regression function reminds us that statistical analysis is usually subject to more than one potential bias. Moreover, the demonstrated interplay between the terms in the decomposition underscores the need to view the biases together rather than in isolation from one another. Finally, the focus on identifiability in Section 6.3 is very relevant, as sometimes not enough is known about the mismeasurement process to yield an identifiable model. The common solution to this problem is to pretend to know more than is justified, in terms of distributional assumptions and parameter values describing the mismeasurement. The result is a model which is identifiable but probably somewhat misspecified. The discussion in 6.3, however, elucidates the value of admitting what is not known via appropriate prior distributions, and proceeding with a nonidentifiable model.

Appendix: Bayes-MCMC Inference

Here we present a primer on the Bayesian paradigm for statistical inference coupled with MCMC algorithms to implement such techniques.

A.1 Bayes Theorem

Say that observable quantities X are thought to be distributed according to a density function $f(x|\theta)$, where θ is an unknown parameter vector. Of course, such use of probability distributions for data given parameters is ubiquitous across various paradigms for statistical inference. In particular, the conditional distribution or density of X given θ is usually referred to as 'the model.' What distinguishes the Bayesian approach, however, is that probability distributions are also used to describe available knowledge about the parameters, both before and after the data are observed. In particular, say the investigator selects a density function $f(\theta)$ to reflect his belief about the value of θ prior to observing the data. This so-called *prior distribution* can be interpreted in a rough sense as follows. If $f(\theta_1) > f(\theta_2)$ for parameter values θ_1 and θ_2, then the investigator views θ values close to θ_1 as being more plausible than θ values close to θ_2, with the ratio $f(\theta_2)/f(\theta_1)$ describing the strength of conviction in this assessment. More formally, prior distributions can be tied to axioms which link rational behaviour and preferences to the existence of *subjective probabilities*. Bernardo and Smith (1994) provide a comprehensive account of this, and other, axiomatic underpinnings of Bayesian analysis.

Armed with the statistical model and the prior distribution, one need only apply the laws of probability to determine the *posterior distribution* of the unknown θ given the observed data $X = x$. This process is summarized as *Bayes theorem*. Further using the common but lazy notation whereby 'f' denotes different densities depending on the context, Bayes theorem can be expressed as

$$f(\theta|x) \quad = \quad \frac{f(x|\theta)f(\theta)}{\int f(x|\theta^*)f(\theta^*)d\theta^*}, \tag{A.1}$$

where the denominator is simply the marginal density of X expressed in terms of the inputted model and prior densities. Under the Bayesian paradigm, (A.1) is a complete encapsulation of knowledge about the unknown θ after seeing the data x. Thus any inferential claims would be based entirely on the posterior distribution.

A useful insight about (A.1) is that the denominator of the right-hand side does not depend on θ. That is, it contributes nothing to the *shape* of the posterior distribution on θ; its only role is to ensure that this distribution is properly normalized. Thus a simpler way to express Bayes theorem is

$$f(\theta|x) \quad \propto \quad f(x|\theta)f(\theta), \tag{A.2}$$

where it must be stressed that the proportionality is as a function of θ. In many situations it is simpler to work with (A.2) and drop multiplicative terms from $f(x|\theta)$ and $f(\theta)$ that do not depend on θ. In some simple problems one can normalize the posterior density by hand as a final step. In problems of more realistic complexity, the required integration cannot be done in closed-form. This necessitates the use of MCMC techniques or some other numerical scheme.

As a simple example of Bayes theorem in action, say an investigator wishes to estimate the prevalence θ of some exposure in a population. Prior to collecting any data, the investigator has some idea about the prevalence from sources such as anecdotal information, studies in similar populations, and scientific common sense. In the present scenario it is convenient to select the prior distribution from the Beta family of distributions. For completeness, the $Beta(c_1, c_2)$ distribution on the unit interval has density function

$$f(\theta|c_1, c_2) \quad = \quad \frac{\Gamma(c_1 + c_2)}{\Gamma(c_1)\Gamma(c_2)}\theta^{c_1-1}(1 - \theta)^{c_2-1}. \tag{A.3}$$

In general when a prior is to be chosen from a parameterized family of distributions, the parameters of this family are termed *hyperparameters*, to distinguish them from the parameters θ in the statistical model for data. Now say the investigator's best prior guess at the prevalence is 0.25, but he acknowledges considerable uncertainty associated with this guess. Upon reflection, he assigns the prior distribution $\theta \sim Beta(2, 4)$. The mode of this distribution coincides with his best guess, as in general the mode of the $Beta(c_1, c_2)$ distribution is $(c_1 - 1)/(c_1 + c_2 - 2)$. But low values of (c_1, c_2) correspond to widely spread distribution, and indeed the plot of the $Beta(2, 4)$ density in Figure A.1 reflects the investigator's considerable *a priori* uncertainty about θ.

Using the standard notion of a sufficient statistic, the observable data can be summarized by the number of the n sampled subjects who are exposed, which we denote by X. Assuming independent sampling from a large population, we have $X|\theta \sim Binomial(n, \theta)$, i.e.

$$f(x|\theta) \quad = \quad \left(\begin{array}{c} n \\ x \end{array} \right) \theta^x(1 - \theta)^{n-x}. \tag{A.4}$$

Applying (A.3) and (A.4) in (A.2) gives the posterior density as

$$f(\theta|x) \propto \theta^{x+c_1-1}(1 - \theta)^{n-x+c_2-1}.$$

Here we can identify that $f(\theta|x)$ is proportional to the $Beta(c_1 + x, c_2 + n - x)$ density, and therefore by normalization $f(\theta|x)$ must in fact be this Beta density function. Thus we have identified the denominator in (A.1) in an implicit manner. In the present context a Beta prior distribution is referred to as a *conjugate prior*, since a Beta prior distribution leads to a Beta posterior distribution.

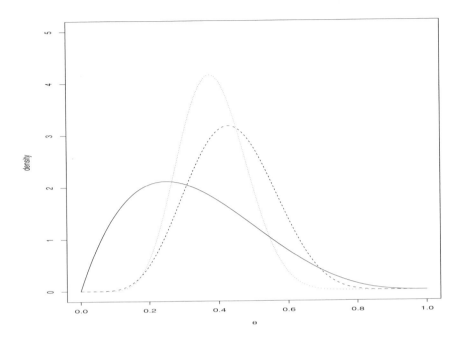

Figure A.1 *Prior and posterior densities of exposure prevalence. The solid curve is the Beta(2,4) prior density. The dashed curve is the Beta(7,9) posterior density after observing 5 out of 10 exposures in a sample from the population. The dotted curve is the Beta(10, 16) posterior density after observing 8 out of 20 exposures in a sample from the population.*

As a concrete example, say that in a sample of $n = 10$ subjects, $x = 5$ are exposed. The combination of these data with the investigator's prior leads to $\theta|x \sim Beta(7, 9)$, the density of which is given in Figure A.1. If three of a further ten sampled subjects are exposed, to yield $x = 8$ and $n = 20$, then $\theta|x \sim Beta(10, 16)$. This posterior density is also plotted in Figure A.1. After both $n = 10$ and $n = 20$ datapoints we see that the posterior mode 'compromises' between the prior mode of 0.25 and the sample proportion x/n, where the latter is the obvious 'data-only' estimate of θ. Note that when $n = 20$ the posterior distribution is narrower, and the prior distribution receives less 'weight' in the compromise than in the $n = 10$ scenario. These are very general phenomena: as the sample size increases the posterior narrows to reflect the accumulating evidence in the data, and the effect of the prior distribution on the posterior distribution diminishes. This is often expressed crudely as the 'data swamp the prior' as the sample size grows.

A.2 Point and Interval Estimates

While an overall summary of the post-data knowledge about an unknown parameter can be conveyed in the form of a posterior density, often specific point and interval estimates are desired. If a point estimate $\hat{\theta}$ of θ is needed, then intuitively one might take $\hat{\theta}$ to be a measure of where the posterior distribution of θ is centred. If the problem at hand yields a symmetric posterior distribution for the parameter in question, then the notion of centre is unambiguous. But say the posterior distribution in question were $\theta|\text{data} \sim Beta(2, 8)$. Then one might consider the posterior mean $\hat{\theta} = 2/10 = 0.2$, the posterior mode $\hat{\theta} = 1/8 = 0.125$, or the posterior median $\hat{\theta} \approx 0.180$ as a formal point estimate of θ. Informally, one might regard the choice between such estimators as a matter of taste. However, basic tenets of *decision theory* have something more precise to say on this matter.

Let $\hat{\theta}(x)$ be an arbitrary estimator of θ based on data x, and let $L(\theta, \hat{\theta})$ be a *loss function* which measures the loss incurred when θ is estimated by $\hat{\theta}$. A fundamental quantity of decision theory is the Bayes risk associated with an estimator and a prior distribution, defined as

$$r = \int \int L(\hat{\theta}(x), \theta) f(x|\theta) f(\theta) dx \; d\theta. \tag{A.5}$$

One way to think of the Bayes risk is as the average loss incurred when estimating θ in repeated experiments, where each experiment consists of 'nature' generating the true parameter value θ from the prior density $f(\theta)$ and then generating the data x from the model density $f(x|\theta)$. This differs from the standard frequentist 'thought experiment' whereby repeated datasets are generated under the same value of θ each time. By changing the order of integration in (A.5) it is easy to see that the estimator $\hat{\theta}(x)$ which minimizes the Bayes risk is

$$\hat{\theta}(x) = \text{argmin}_a \int L(\theta, a) f(\theta|x) d\theta, \tag{A.6}$$

where the integral on the right-hand side is the so called *posterior risk* associated with estimate or 'action' a. The fact that the optimal estimator is necessarily based on the posterior distribution via (A.6) is regarded as a sense in which Bayesian analysis is the optimal procedure in light of a prior weighting of the parameter space. Moreover, if one selects a loss function then there is no longer ambiguity about how to obtain a point estimate from the posterior distribution. For instance, it is easy to verify that if squared-error loss is chosen, so that $L(\hat{\theta}, \theta) = (\hat{\theta} - \theta)^2$, then the particular estimator which minimizes (A.6) is the posterior mean, $\hat{\theta}(x) = E(\theta|x)$. Similarly, under absolute error loss, $L(\hat{\theta}, \theta) = |\hat{\theta} - \theta|$, (A.6) is minimized by the posterior median $\hat{\theta} = med(\theta|x)$.

Often interval estimates are also desired. This is particularly easy under the Bayesian paradigm, as the posterior distribution immediately conveys a sense of how likely it is that the parameter in question lies in a specific interval.

As a formal definition, any interval which is assigned probability $(1 - \alpha)$ by the posterior distribution of θ is called a $100(1 - \alpha)\%$ credible interval for θ. Note that the interpretation of a Bayesian credible interval is more direct than that of a frequentist confidence interval. Say, for instance, that (a, b) is a 95% credible interval for θ. Then it is legitimate to state the probability of θ lying between a and b given the observed data is 0.95. On the other hand, it is standard to caution that frequentist confidence intervals cannot be given this direct interpretation. The best that can be said is that on average such intervals contain the true parameter nineteen times out of twenty.

Of course for a given posterior distribution one can construct many different $100(1 - \alpha)\%$ credible intervals. The two most common and intuitive choices are the equal-tailed credible interval and the highest posterior density (HPD) credible interval. As its name suggests, the $100(1 - \alpha)\%$ equal-tailed credible interval has the $\alpha/2$ and $1 - \alpha/2$ quantiles of the posterior distribution $\theta|X$ as its endpoints. On the other hand, the $100(1 - \alpha)\%$ HPD credible interval consists of all values of θ for which $f(\theta|x) > c$, where c is chosen to ensure that the interval does have posterior probability $1 - \alpha$. In some situations involving a multimodal posterior distribution this definition could lead to an HPD region (say a union of disjoint intervals) rather than an interval. In the common situation of a unimodal posterior distribution, however, an interval is guaranteed. An important and easily verified property is that the $100(1-\alpha)\%$ HPD credible interval is the shortest possible $100(1 - \alpha)\%$ credible interval.

It is often overlooked, but credible intervals do have a repeated sampling interpretation. As introduced with the notion of Bayes risk, consider repeated sampling whereby each sample is obtained by first generating θ from the prior distribution and then generating data x from the model distribution for $X|\theta$. It is trivial to establish that with respect to such sampling there is probability $(1 - \alpha)$ that a $100(1 - \alpha)\%$ credible interval for θ based on the X will actually contain θ. In this sense a credible interval is a weaker notion than a confidence interval which has the repeated sampling interpretation regardless of how the true θ values are generated. Of course in many practical problems it is not possible to construct exact confidence intervals, whereas the construction of credible intervals is entirely general.

A.3 Markov Chain Monte Carlo

In many problems the combination of the model distribution for data given parameters and the prior distribution for parameters leads to a complicated posterior distribution for parameters given data. By complicated we mean a nonstandard distribution under which it is hard to compute probabilities and expectations. More definitely, often there is no closed-form solution for the integral in the denominator of (A.1). The problem becomes particularly acute as the number of unknown parameters grows, as numerical integration techniques suffer from a *curse of dimensionality*. Until about 1990, these numerical difficulties severely limited the range of applications for Bayesian analysis.

The Bayesian approach to statistics underwent a quantum leap with the realization that computational techniques originating in statistical physics and chemistry had great potential for determining posterior distributions arising in complex models with many parameters. The first algorithm to be applied in statistical contexts was the *Gibbs sampler* (Gelfand and Smith 1990, Gelfand *et al.* 1990), though this was soon realized to be just one specialization of the *Metropolis-Hastings* (MH) algorithm (Metropolis *et al.* 1953; Hastings 1970), and that other specializations were also very promising. Collectively the algorithms in question tend to be referred to as *Markov Chain Monte Carlo* (MCMC) algorithms. There are now numerous general references on MCMC methods, including the books of Gammerman (1997) and Chen, Shao, and Ibrahim (2000).

The broad idea is that one way to compute quantities associated with a particular *target distribution* is to simulate a large Monte Carlo sample of realizations from this distribution. Then probabilities and expectations under the target distribution can be approximated by analogous quantities in the Monte Carlo sample. Generally, if the Monte Carlo sample is comprised of m realizations, then the approximation error gets smaller at a rate of $m^{-1/2}$. When the target distribution is the posterior distribution over θ arising from a particular dataset, one can evaluate the unnormalized version of the target density (A.2) at any given θ value. The challenge is to use such evaluations to draw a Monte Carlo sample from the target distribution.

Usually with a complicated likelihood function and prior density one cannot (a) simulate independent and identically distributed realizations from the posterior distribution, or even (b) simulate *dependent* but identically distributed realizations from the posterior distribution. What MCMC methods can do, however, is (c) simulate from a *Markov chain* having the posterior distribution as its stationary distribution. Theory dictates that under weak regularity conditions a Markov chain will converge quickly to its stationary distribution, so in fact (c) is almost as good as (b). One can simulate from the Markov chain and then discard the first portion of sampled values as a 'burn-in' period which allows the chain to converge. The remaining sampled values are then treated as (b), a dependent sample from the posterior distribution. In general one can still estimate features of a target distribution with a dependent rather than independent sample from the distribution. However, this estimation becomes more inefficient as the strength of the serial dependence in the Markov chain increases. Hence there are two different concerns about how well a particular MCMC algorithm works in learning the features of a particular posterior distribution: is convergence to the posterior distribution fast, and does the sampler *mix* or move around the possible parameter values rapidly. That is, is the dependence mild enough for the Monte Carlo sample to yield good estimates of posterior distribution features.

The MH algorithm has a remarkably simple form. Say the target density of interest for a vector θ of dimension p is $s(\theta)$, and let $t(b|a)$ be a conditional distribution from which we can simulate a *candidate state* b given a *current state* a. We generate our Markov chain $\theta^{(1)}, \ldots, \theta^{(m)}$ by setting $\theta^{(1)}$ to have some arbitrary value, and then iterating the following three-part updating scheme to generate $\theta^{(i+1)}$ given $\theta^{(i)}$.

1. Simulate a candidate value θ^* from the conditional density $t(\theta^*|\theta^{(i)})$.
2. Compute the acceptance probability

$$pr \;=\; \min\left\{ \frac{s(\theta^*)}{s(\theta^{(i)})}\,\frac{t(\theta^{(i)}|\theta^*)}{t(\theta^*|\theta^{(i)})}, 1 \right\}.$$

3. Simulate a 'biased coin flip' to set

$$\theta^{(i+1)} \;=\; \begin{cases} \theta^* & \text{with probability } pr, \\ \theta^{(i)} & \text{with probability } 1 - pr. \end{cases}$$

Note that only an unnormalized expression for the target density is required to implement the MH algorithm, as the acceptance probability depends on s only through the ratio of $s(\theta^*)/s(\theta^{(i)})$. Clearly when the target density is a posterior density this ratio is $\{f(y|\theta^*)f(\theta^*)\}/\{f(y|\theta^{(i)})f(\theta^{(i)})\}$, which can be evaluated regardless of whether the posterior density can be normalized in closed-form.

It it quite straightforward to show that the Metropolis-Hastings update does have the target density as its stationary distribution. That is, if $\theta^{(i)} \sim s()$ then $\theta^{(i+1)} \sim s()$. Markov chain theory then dictates that under weak regularity conditions the distribution of $\theta^{(i)}$ converges quickly to $s()$ as i increases. Much of the requisite Markov chain theory is made quite accessible by Robert and Casella (1999). We emphasize that here 'quick' convergence means at an exponential rate, so that formal measures of the distance between the actual distribution of $\theta^{(i)}$ and the target distribution behave like $\exp(-ci)$ for some $c > 0$, as opposed to the slow $i^{-1/2}$ convergence of most limiting theorems in statistics. Thus after allowing m^* burn-in iterations one can estimate target distribution features with corresponding sample features of $\theta^{(m^*+1)}, \ldots, \theta^{(m^*+m)}$. An important aspect of MCMC is choosing m^* and m to be large enough to compute target distribution features with desired accuracy.

The MH algorithm is exceedingly general in that one can choose any conditional density $t(\cdot|\cdot)$ from which to generate candidates. In practice, however, one must make intelligent choices in order to get reasonable performance. Often it is necessary to reduce a high-dimensional problem to a series of one-dimensional problems, by generating candidate vectors which differ from the current vector in only one component.

The Gibbs sampler is such an algorithm that is useful when the joint target distribution on a vector θ does not have a standard form but does yield standard forms for the distribution of each single component given the other components. The target distribution of a single component given all the other components is referred to as the *full conditional* distribution of that component. It is easy to check that generating a candidate by sampling from the full conditional for one component while leaving the other components unchanged leads to an acceptance probability of one in the MH algorithm. Thus candidates are never rejected. To be more specific, if all three full conditionals for

$\theta = (\theta_1, \theta_2, \theta_3)$ are standard distributions, then one complete Gibbs sampler iteration from $\theta^{(i)}$ to $\theta^{(i+1)}$ is completed as

1. simulate $\theta_1^{(i+1)}$ from $s(\theta_1 | \theta_2 = \theta_2^{(i)}, \theta_3 = \theta_3^{(i)})$,

2. simulate $\theta_2^{(i+1)}$ from $s(\theta_2 | \theta_1 = \theta_1^{(i+1)}, \theta_3 = \theta_3^{(i)})$,

3. simulate $\theta_3^{(i+1)}$ from $s(\theta_3 | \theta_1 = \theta_1^{(i+1)}, \theta_2 = \theta_2^{(i+1)})$.

The obvious drawback to the Gibbs sampler is that some full conditionals may be very difficult to simulate from. While there are some fairly general approaches to so doing (see, for instance, Gilks and Wild 1992; Gilks, Best and Tan 1995), sometimes candidate generation schemes which do not rely on sampling the full conditional distributions are necessary. One of the simplest such schemes is the *random-walk* MH algorithm. If the strategy of reducing to one-dimensional updates is followed, a candidate θ^* is obtained from $\theta^{(i)}$ by adding 'noise' to one component of θ^*. By generating the noise from a distribution which is symmetric about zero, we obtain the simplification that $t(\theta^* | \theta^{(i)}) = t(\theta^{(i)} | \theta^*)$. Consequently the acceptance probability will depend only on the ratio $s(\theta^*)/s(\theta^{(i)})$, making it very simple to implement this algorithm. Typically the primary challenge is 'tuning' the variation in the noise distribution. In particular, say that when the j-th component of θ is updated the candidate is formed via $\theta_j^* \sim N\left(\theta_j^{(i)}, \sigma_j^2\right)$. One must then select values of $\sigma_1, \ldots, \sigma_p$ which yield reasonable performance from the algorithm, where σ_j is often referred to as the *jump size* for the θ_j update. To large extent this is a trial-and-error process, though there is some useful guidance in the literature to which we refer shortly.

Perhaps the vast majority of MCMC-based inference done in practice uses some combination of the Gibbs sampler and the random walk MH algorithms, primarily because they are simple to understand and implement. On the other hand, more specialized and powerful MH algorithms are sometimes needed. Numerous such algorithms have been investigated, such as the hybrid algorithm which uses extra information in the form of derivatives of the posterior density, and various algorithms which introduce auxiliary variables in an attempt to more freely traverse the parameter space. Also, parameter reparameterizations which tend to improve MCMC performance have been studied. Recent books which cover more specialized algorithms include Chen, Shao, and Ibrahim (2000), and Liu (2001).

To get some intuition for MCMC we try the Gibbs sampler and random walk MH algorithms on a simple bivariate normal target distribution, namely

$$\begin{pmatrix} \theta_1 \\ \theta_2 \end{pmatrix} \sim N\left(\begin{pmatrix} 0 \\ 0 \end{pmatrix}\begin{pmatrix} 1 & \rho \\ \rho & 1 \end{pmatrix}\right).$$

Of course this is an artificial example, as it is trivial to sample directly from the target distribution. Nonetheless, we will be able to develop some intuition about the algorithms in this test case.

Figure A.2 gives traceplots of θ_1 for 500 iterations of the Gibbs sampler and of the random-walk MH algorithm with three different jump sizes

($\sigma = 0.25$, $\sigma = 1.25$, $\sigma = 3$). In fact two different target distributions are considered ($\rho = 0.5$, $\rho = 0.9$). In each case the initial state is taken to be $(\theta_1^{(1)}, \theta_2^{(1)}) = (10, 10)$, which of course is very far from where the target distribution is concentrated. All four algorithms appear to mix better for the $\rho = 0.5$ target distribution than for the $\rho = 0.9$ target distribution. In fact this is a very general phenomenon: MCMC algorithms tend to perform less well when the target distribution involves stronger dependencies. For both target distributions the Gibbs sampler outperforms the random-walk MH algorithm, in terms of both faster convergence and better mixing. This is not surprising given that the Gibbs sampler relies on more knowledge about the target distribution in the form of the full conditional distributions. Thus Gibbs sampling tends to be favoured whenever full conditional distributions have standard forms.

It is clear from Figure A.2 that the performance of the random walk MH algorithm depends quite strongly on the choice of jump size. Intuitively, the jump size will correlate negatively with the *acceptance rate*, i.e., the proportion of the iterations at which the candidate state is accepted. A small jump size will correspond to small differences between the target density at the current and candidate states, so that small values of the acceptance probability are unlikely. Conversely, a large jump size will tend to generate candidate states which miss the region where the target distribution is concentrated. The form of the acceptance probability indicates that such candidates are very likely to be rejected. The acceptance rates given in Figure A.2 do indeed decrease as the jump size increases.

On the face of it, a high acceptance rate seems good, as it suggests the sampler is unlikely to get stuck at the same value for a number of successive iterations. However, this comes at the cost of only making very small moves. Thus with a jump size of $\sigma = 0.25$ (yielding acceptance rates of 85% when $\rho = 0.5$ and 78% when $\rho = 0.9$) the algorithm is seen to converge slowly and mix poorly in Figure A.2. The figure indicates that the tradeoff of bigger jumps ($\sigma = 1.25$) at the cost of lower acceptance rates (51% when $\rho = 0.5$ and 33% when $\rho = 0.9$) seems worthwhile. That is, both faster convergence and better mixing are evident. Intuitively, however, a very low acceptance rate does not seem appealing, as this would entail the value of θ not changing at most iterations. This is supported by the poor 'boxy' mixing with a jump size of $\sigma = 3$ (and acceptance rates of 24% when $\rho = 0.5$ and 13% when $\rho = 0.9$). Indeed, theoretical work of Roberts, Gelman, and Gilks (1997) supports the notion that the random-walk MH algorithm works best at a mid-range acceptance rate, with common practice being to select jump sizes by trial-and-error in order to obtain an acceptance rate perhaps in the range of 35% to 60%. Roberts and Rosenthal (2001) provide an accessible review of work on the so called 'optimal scaling' of MH algorithms.

As a final comment about the example, note that a particular jump size yields a lower acceptance rate when ρ is larger. Since we are applying the random walk MH algorithm in a 'one-component at a time' fashion, the relevant

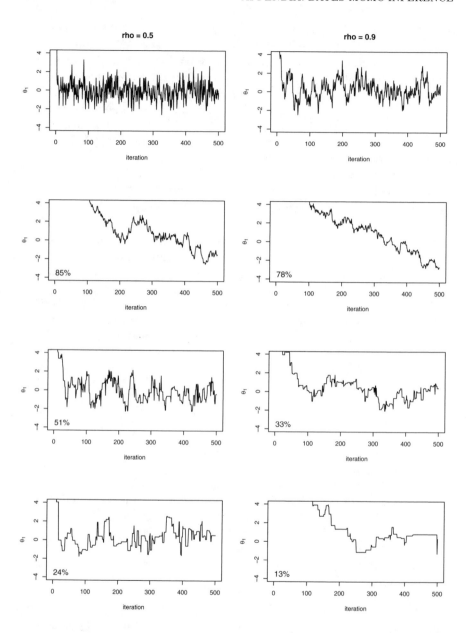

Figure A.2 *MCMC algorithms applied to a bivariate normal target distribution. Each panel plots the sampled values of θ_1 against iteration, for 500 iterations of the algorithm. The left panels correspond to a $\rho = 0.5$ target, while the right panels correspond to $\rho = 0.9$. From top to bottom the rows correspond to different algorithms: the Gibbs sampler, and the random walk MH algorithm with jump sizes $\sigma = 0.25$, $\sigma = 1.25$, $\sigma = 3$. For the random walk MH algorithm the acceptance rate is given in the bottom left corner of each panel.*

variation in the posterior distribution is the variation in the full conditional distributions. That is, the update to the j-th component of θ can be regarded as an update with the j-th full conditional distribution as the target distribution. Since larger ρ corresponds to narrower full conditionals in our example, a fixed jump size σ can be thought of as becoming effectively larger as ρ increases.

Here we have examined the MCMC output very informally, making qualitative statements about how good the output is, and consequently how well it might represent the target distribution. In fact there is a large literature on more formal assessments. Much of this revolves around *convergence diagnostics*, which attempt to determine empirically how many burn-in iterations are required. The first and perhaps most popular diagnostic is that of Gelman and Rubin (1992). It involves a simple scheme based on implementing multiple chains and comparing between and within chain variation. Much of the later suggestions are more technical, involving more sophisticated Markov chain theory. Many of the suggested schemes are reviewed by Mengersen, Robert and Guihenneuc-Jouyaux (1999).

As a further point about MCMC output for a given posterior distribution, usually the actual computation of point and interval estimates is carried out in the intuitively obvious way. For instance, say that post burn-in output $\theta^{(1)}, \ldots, \theta^{(m)}$ is obtained when the target distribution is a posterior distribution for θ given observed data. And say the scalar parameter $\psi = g(\theta)$ is of interest. Then the sample mean or median of $g(\theta^{(1)}), \ldots, g(\theta^{(m)})$ could be reported as the posterior mean or median of ψ. Similarly, appropriate sample quantiles could be reported as an equal-tailed credible interval for ψ, while the computation of HPD credible intervals is slightly more involved. We emphasize that these are actually *approximations* to posterior quantities which involve numerical error, often referred to as Monte Carlo error or simulation error. The exact values of posterior quantities would only be obtained in the large m limit of infinite Monte Carlo sample size. However, typically the approximation error can be made very small in relation to the actual statistical uncertainty at play. With a careful choice of MCMC algorithm and a sufficiently large m, for instance, the difference between the Monte Carlo approximation and the actual posterior mean of a parameter can be made as small as desired in relation to the difference between the actual posterior mean and the true value of the parameter. Following along these lines, sometimes it is relevant to report a simulation standard error, perhaps on the basis of the variation in estimates over multiple Markov chain runs. Then the relevant check would be whether the simulation standard error is indeed small in relation to say the posterior standard deviation of the parameter in question.

Finally, often one wishes to convey the shape of marginal posterior distributions, either instead of, or in addition to, formal point and interval estimates. With respect to the notation above, an obvious approximation to the posterior marginal distribution of ψ is a histogram of $g(\theta^{(1)}), \ldots, g(\theta^{(m)})$. If the inherent coarseness of a histogram is not appealing, then a smooth approximation to the marginal posterior density can be obtained by applying kernel density estimation to the sampled values. As a default in this book we have used kernel density estimation with the general-purpose bandwidth suggested by Silverman (1986). On occasion, however, it is necessary to increase the bandwidth by hand, in order to obtain a plausibly smooth approximation to the posterior marginal density.

A.4 Prior Selection

A necessity with any Bayesian analysis is the specification of a prior distribution for the unknown parameters. Depending on one's views and the nature of the problem at hand, this can be viewed as a strength or a weakness of the Bayesian approach. A 'pure' Bayesian approach dictates that the prior distribution is strictly a representation of the investigator's belief about the parameters before seeing the data, and a sizeable literature describes *elicitation procedures* to capture beliefs in the form of probability distributions. Some recent references on elicitation include Kadane and Wolfson (1998), and O'Hagan (1998). It is the case, however, that most Bayesian analysis done in practice makes limited or no use of formal elicitation procedures. This is probably because meaningful elicitation is viewed as too difficult, particularly when the number of unknown parameters is large. Instead, often computational convenience and a desire to *not* impart strong prior views into the analysis are primary factors in the selection of a prior distribution.

As a simple example, say $X_1, \ldots, X_n$ are independent and identically distributed from a $N(\mu, \sigma^2)$ distribution. For computational expedience one might consider a prior distribution of the form

$$\mu | \sigma^2 \ \sim \ N\left(\tilde{\mu}, \frac{\sigma^2}{k_1}\right),$$

$$\sigma^2 \ \sim \ IG\left(\frac{k_2}{2}, \frac{k_2 \tilde{\sigma}^2}{2}\right),$$

where N and IG denote *normal* and *inverse-gamma* distributions respectively. Note that $(\tilde{\mu}, \tilde{\sigma}^2, k_1, k_2)$ are hyperparameters that must be specified. In particular, $\tilde{\mu}$ and $\tilde{\sigma}^2$ can be regarded as prior guesses at the parameter values, particularly as an $IG(a, b)$ distribution is roughly centred at b/a. The role of k_1 and k_2 is less clear, but we will see momentarily that intuitive meanings can be ascribed to these hyperparameters. Another curious feature of this prior is that the two parameters are *not* independent *a priori*. The rationale for this derives more from the resultant interpretability of the posterior distribution than from an inherent sense that prior beliefs about the two parameters ought to be correlated. An important feature is that the prior is *conditionally conjugate*, in the sense that $\mu | \sigma^2, x$ has a normal distribution while $\sigma^2 | \mu, x$ has an inverse gamma distribution. Consequently, it is trivial to implement Gibbs sampling in such a scenario, and in more complicated variants as well.

More specifically, the posterior full conditional distributions are identified as

$$\mu | \sigma^2, x \quad \sim \quad N\left\{\left(\frac{n}{n+k_1}\right)\bar{x} + \left(\frac{k_1}{k_1+n}\right)\tilde{\mu}, \frac{\sigma^2}{n+k_1}\right\} \qquad (A.7)$$

and

$$\sigma^2 | \mu, x \quad \sim \quad IG\left(\frac{n+k_2}{2}, \frac{ns^2 + k_2\tilde{\sigma}^2}{2}\right), \qquad (A.8)$$

where $\bar{x}$ and s^2 denote the sample mean and variance. These forms suggest k_1 and k_2 be interpreted as *effective sample sizes* for the prior distributions of μ and σ^2 respectively. This is evident from examining both the centre and variation of the distributions (A.7) and (A.8). We see that both distributions are centred at linear combinations of a sample-based estimate and the prior guess, with the former having weight $n/(n+k_j)$ and the latter having weight $k_j/(k_j+n)$. Moreover, the variation in both distributions declines as $1/(n+k_j)$. Thus the information content in prior (A.7) can be viewed as equivalent to k_1 observed data points, and the content of (A.8) as equivalent to k_2 observed data points. A relatively common approach is to choose $k_1 = 1$ and $k_2 = 1$, to ensure the prior gets little weight compared to the data. Such a choice has been termed a *unit-information prior* by Kass and Wasserman (1995), who investigate some theoretical aspects of using such priors. Thinking about prior specification in terms of prior guesses and effective sample sizes is a pragmatic way of obtaining a reasonable prior distribution without an extensive elicitation process.

No matter what degree of comfort one has in a particular prior, it seems reasonable to ask how posterior inferences would change if the prior were changed. Indeed, some would argue that such *prior sensitivity* analysis is a vital part of the Bayesian approach. Thus it is relatively common to see an analysis repeated with a few different choices of prior distribution. As well, more formal mathematical techniques can be used to quantify the sensitivity of a Bayesian inference to the choice of prior. Ríos-Insua and Ruggeri (2000) provide a recent overview of such techniques.

A.5 MCMC and Unobserved Structure

Much of the advantage of MCMC-based inference arises in problems where succinct expression of the model distribution for data given parameters, or the prior distribution for parameters, is problematic. In many problems there is inherent unobserved structure that in some sense lies between the observed data and the unknown parameters. Outside the realm of mismeasured variables, examples of such unobserved quantities include the random effects in a variance components model, the actual failure times for censored observations in a lifetime data model, the unobserved continuous responses linked to observed binary responses in a probit model, and the values of missing covariates in a regression model.

To be more specific, consider a model involving random effects. Let A denote the data to be observed, let B be the unobservable random effects, and let C be the fixed effects and variance components. Traditionally one would regard only C as unknown parameters, so that Bayesian inference would be based on the distribution of $C|A$. On the face of it one would require a model distribution for $(A|C)$ and a prior distribution for C in order to obtain this posterior distribution. However, depending on the form of the random effects model it may not be possible to determine the distribution of $(A|C)$ explicitly. An appealing alternative is to consider a joint distribution over all quantities, in the form of $f(a, b, c) = f(a|b, c)f(b|c)f(c)$. Then Bayes theorem and MCMC allow one to obtain a posterior sample from $(B, C|A)$, the joint distribution of random effects and unknown parameters given observed data. Then trivially the sampled C values comprise a sample from the distribution of $(C|A)$, enabling the desired inferences. Simply put, MCMC is very effective at exploiting complex hierarchical structure in models, with the requisite integration carried out behind the scenes.

Another example that falls into the framework above is models where the response variable can be represented via latent structure. For instance, the binary responses A in a probit model can be viewed as arising from thresholding of unobserved continuous responses B, with the relevant parameters again denoted by C. While there is no closed-form for the posterior distribution of parameters C given data A, there is a closed-form for the posterior distribution of parameters C given A and B. Thus this full conditional distribution is readily sampled, as are the full conditionals for A and B. In essence MCMC makes this intractable problem tractable, as noted by Carlin and Polson (1992), and Albert and Chib (1993).

In a slightly more elaborate example of direct relevance to this book, let A be the mismeasured values of an explanatory variable, let B be the response variable values, let C be the true but unobservable values of the explanatory variable, and let D be the unknown parameters involved. Ultimately one wishes to base inferences on the distribution of $(D|A, B)$; however it may be impossible to get an explicit form for $(A, B|D)$ in order to apply Bayes theorem directly. Instead, one can use MCMC to sample from $(C, D|A, B)$, given that the distributions of $(A|B, C, D)$, $(B|C, D)$, $(C|D)$, and D are available. As above, an ability to sample from $(C, D|A, B)$ automatically implies an ability to sample from the desired distribution of $(D|A, B)$. Again MCMC can be very effective at exploiting the model structure to get at the desired but complicated distributions via simpler distributions.

References

Adcock, R.J. (1877). Note on the method of least squares. *Analyst* **4**, 183-184.

Adcock, R.J. (1878). A problem in least squares. *Analyst* **5**, 53-54.

Albert, J.H. and Chib, S. (1993), Bayesian analysis of binary and polychotomous response data. *Journal of the American Statistical Association* **88**, 669-679.

Armstrong, B.G., Whittemore, A.S., and Howe, G.R. (1989). Analysis of case-control data with covariate measurement error: application to diet and colon cancer. *Statistics in Medicine* **8**, 1151-1163.

Armstrong, B.K., White, E., and Saracci, R. (1992). *Principles of Exposure Measurement in Epidemiology.* Oxford University Press, Oxford.

Band, P.R., Spinelli, J.J., Threlfall, W.J., Fang, R., Le, N.D. and Gallagher, R.P. (1999). Identification of occupational cancer risks in British Columbia— Part I: Methodology, descriptive results, and analysis of cancer risks by cigarette smoking categories of 15,463 incident cancer cases. *Journal of Occupational and Environmental Medicine* **41**, 224-232.

Barron, B.A. (1977). The effects of misclassification on the estimation of relative risk. *Biometrics* **33**, 414-418.

Bashir, S.A. and Duffy, S.W. (1997). The correction of risk estimates for measurement error. *Annals of Epidemiology* **7**, 154-164.

Bashir, S.A., Duffy, S.W., and Qizilbash, N. (1997). Repeat measurements of case-control data: corrections for measurement error in a study of ischaemic stroke and haemostatic factors. *International Journal of Epidemiology* **26**, 64-70.

Begg, M.D. and Lagakos, S. (1992). Effects of mismodelling on tests of association based on logistic regression models. *Annals of Statistics* **20**, 1929-1952.

Begg, M.D. and Lagakos, S. (1993). Loss of efficiency caused by omitting covariates and misspecifying exposure in logistic regression models. *Journal of the American Statistical Association* **88**, 166-170.

Bernardo, J.M. and Smith, A.F.M. (1994). *Bayesian Theory.* Wiley, New York.

Berry, S.A., Carroll, R.J., and Ruppert, D. (2002). Bayesian smoothing and regression splines for measurement error problems. *Journal of the American Statistical Association* **97**, 160-69.

Birkett, N.J. (1992). Effect of nondifferential misclassification on estimates of odds ratios with multiple levels of exposure. *American Journal of Epidemiology* **136**, 356-362.

Brenner, H. (1996). How independent are multiple 'independent' diagnostic classifications? *Statistics in Medicine* **15**, 1377-1386.

Bross, I. (1954). Misclassification in 2 × 2 tables. *Biometrics* **10**, 478-486.

Brown, J., Kreiger, N., Darlington, G.A., and Sloan, M. (2001). Misclassification of exposure: coffee as a surrogate for caffeine intake. *American Journal of Epidemiology* **153**, 815-820.

Buonaccorsi, J.P. (1990). Double sampling for exact values in the normal discriminant model with application to binary regression. *Communications in Statistics A* **19**, 4569-4586.

Carlin, B.P. and Polson, N.G. (1992). Monte Carlo Bayesian methods for discrete regression models and categorical time series. In *Bayesian Statistics 4* (J.M. Bernardo, J.O. Berger, A.P. Dawid, and A.F.M. Smith, eds.). Oxford University Press, Oxford, pp. 577-568.

Carroll, R.J. (1997). Surprising effects of measurement error on an aggregate data estimation. *Biometrika* **84**, 231-234.

Carroll, R.J., Roeder, K., and Wasserman, L. (1999). Flexible parametric measurement error models. *Biometrics* **55**, 44-54.

Carroll, R.J., Ruppert, D., and Stefanski, L.A. (1995). *Measurement Error in Nonlinear Models.* Chapman and Hall, Boca Raton.

Carroll, R.J., Spiegelman, C.H., Lan, K.K.G., Bailey, K.T., and Abbott, R.D. (1984). On errors-in-variables for binary regression models. *Biometrika* **71**, 19-25.

Carroll, R.J. and Stefanski, L.A. (1990). Approximate quasilikelihood estimation in problems with surrogate predictors. *Journal of the American Statistical Association* **85**, 652-663.

Chen, M.H., Shao, Q.M., and Ibrahim, J.G. (2000). *Monte Carlo Methods in Bayesian Computation.* Springer, New York.

Chen, T.T. (1989). A review of methods for misclassified categorical data in epidemiology. *Statistics in Medicine* **8**, 1095–1106.

Cochran, W.G. (1968). Errors of measurement in statistics. *Technometrics* **10**, 637-666.

Cook, J. and Stefanski, L.A. (1995). A simulation extrapolation method for parametric measurement error models. *Journal of the American Statistical Association* **89**, 1414-1328.

Copeland, K.T., Checkoway, H., McMichael, A.J., and Holbrook, R.H. (1977). Bias due to the misclassification of relative risk. *American Journal of Epidemiology* **105**, 488-495.

Crouch, E.A.C. and Spiegelman, D. (1990). The evaluation of integrals of the form $\int_{-\infty}^{\infty} f(t) \exp(-t^2) dt$: applications to logistic-normal models. *Journal of the American Statistical Association* **85**, 464-467.

Dawber, T.R., Kannel, W.B., and Lyell, L.P. (1963). An approach to longitudinal studies in a community: the Framingham study. *Annals of the New York Academy of Science* **107**, 539-556.

Dawid, A.P. (1979). Conditional independence in statistical theory (with discussion). *Journal of the Royal Statistical Society B* **41**, 1-31.

Dellaportas, P. and Stephens, D.A. (1995). Bayesian analysis of errors-in-variables regression models. *Biometrics* **51**, 1085-1095.

Delpizzo, V. and Borghes, J.L. (1995). Exposure measurement errors, risk estimate and statistical power in case-control studies using dichotomous analysis of a continuous exposure variable. *International Journal of Epidemiology* **24**, 851-862.

Dempster, A.P., Laird, N.M., and Rubin, D.B. (1977). Maximum likelihood from incomplete data via the EM algorithm. *Journal of the Royal Statistical Society B* **39**, 1-38.

Dendukuri, N. and Joseph, L. (2001). Bayesian approaches to modelling the conditional dependence between multiple diagnostic tests. *Biometrics* **57**, 158-167.

Dosemeci, M., Wacholder, S., and Lubin, J.H. (1990). Does nondifferential misclassification of exposure always bias a true effect toward the null value? *American Journal of Epidemiology* **132**, 746-748.

Drews, C.D., Flanders, W.D., and Kosinski, A.S. (1993). Use of two data sources to estimate odds-ratios in case-control studies. *Epidemiology* **4**, 327-335.

Durbin, J. (1954). Errors-in-variables. *International Statistical Review* **22**, 23-32.

Evans, M., Guttman, I., Haitovsky, Y., and Swartz, T.B. (1995). Bayesian analysis of binary data subject to misclassification. In *Bayesian Statistics and Econometrics: Essays in Honor of Arnold Zellner* (D. Berry, K.M. Chaloner, and J. Geweke, eds.). Wiley, New York. pp. 67-77.

Evans, M. and Swartz, T.B. (2000). *Approximating integrals via Monte Carlo and deterministic methods.* Oxford University Press, Oxford.

Flegal, K.M., Keyl, P.M., and Nieto, F.J. (1991). Differential misclassification arising from nondifferential errors in exposure measurement. *American Journal of Epidemiology* **134**, 1233-1244.

Fryback, D.G. (1978). Bayes' theorem and conditional nonindependence of data in medical diagnosis. *Biomedical Research* **11**, 423-434.

Fuller, W.A. (1987). *Measurement Error Models.* Wiley, New York.

Gammerman, D. (1997). *Stochastic Simulation for Bayesian Inference.* Chapman and Hall, Boca Raton.

Gelfand, A.E., Hills, S.E., Racine-Poon, A., and Smith, A.F.M. (1990). Illustration of Bayesian inference in normal data models using Gibbs sampling. *Journal of the American Statistical Association* **85**, 972-985.

Gelfand, A.E., and Smith, A.F.M. (1990). Sampling-based approaches to calculating marginal densities. *Journal of the American Statistical Association* **85**, 398-409.

Gelfand, A.E. and Sahu, S.K. (1999). Identifiability, improper priors, and Gibbs sampling for generalized linear models. *Journal of the American Statistical Association* **94**, 247-253.

Gelman, A. and Rubin, D.B. (1992). Inference from iterative simulation using multiple sequences (with discussion). *Statistical Science* **7**, 457-511.

Gentle, J.E. (1998). *Numerical Linear Algebra for Applications in Statistics.* Springer, New York.

Gilks, W.R. and Roberts, G.O. (1996). Strategies for improving MCMC. In *Markov Chain Monte Carlo in Practice* (W.R. Gilks, S. Richardson, and D.J. Spiegelhalter, eds.). Chapman and Hall, Boca Raton.

Gilks, W.R. and Wild, P. (1992). Adaptive rejection sampling for Gibbs sampling. *Applied Statistics* **41**, 337-348.

Gilks, W.R., Best, N.G., and Tan, K.K.C. (1995). Adaptive rejection Metropolis sampling within Gibbs sampling. *Applied Statistics* **44**, 455- 472.

Gleser, L.J. (1990). Improvements of the naive approach to estimation in nonlinear errors-in-variables regression models. In *Statistical Analysis of Measurement Error Models and Application* (P.J. Brown and W.A. Fuller, eds.). American Mathematical Society, Providence.

Goldberg, J.D. (1975). The effect of misclassification on the bias in the difference between two proportions and the relative odds in the fourfold table. *Journal of the American Statistical Association* **70**, 561-567.

Green, P.J. (1995). Reversible jump Markov chain Monte Carlo computation and Bayesian model determination. *Biometrika* **82**, 711-732.

Greenland, S. (1980). The effect of misclassification in the presence of covariates. *American Journal of Epidemiology* **112**, 564-569.

Greenland, S. (1988). Statistical uncertainty due to misclassification: implications for validation substudies. *Journal of Clinical Epidemiology* **41**, 1167-1174.

Greenland, S. and Kleinbaum, D.G. (1983). Correcting for misclassification in two-way tables and matched-pair studies. *International Journal of Epidemiology* **12**, 93-97.

Gustafson, P. (1997). Large hierarchical Bayesian analysis of multivariate survival data. *Biometrics* **53**, 230-242.

Gustafson, P. (1998). Flexible Bayesian modelling for survival data. *Lifetime Data Analysis* **4**, 281-299.

Gustafson, P. (2002a). On the simultaneous effects of model misspecification and errors-in-variables. *Canadian Journal of Statistics* **30**, 463-474.

Gustafson, P. (2002b). On model expansion, model contraction, identifiability, and prior information: two illustrative scenarios involving mismeasured variables. Technical Report 203, Department of Statistics, University of British Columbia.

Gustafson, P. and Le, N.D. (2002). Comparing the effects of continuous and discrete covariate mismeasurement, with emphasis on the dichtomization of mismeasured predictors. *Biometrics* **58**, 878-887.

Gustafson, P., Le, N.D., and Saskin, R. (2001). Case-control analysis with partial knowledge of exposure misclassification probabilities. *Biometrics* **57**, 598-609.

Gustafson, P., Le, N.D., and Vallée, M. (2000). Parametric Bayesian analysis of case-control data with imprecise exposure measurements. *Statistics and Probability Letters* **47**, 357-363.

Gustafson, P., Le, N.D., and Vallée, M. (2002). A Bayesian approach to case-control studies with errors in covariables. *Biostatistics* **3**, 229-243.

Gustafson, P. and Wasserman, L. (1996). Comment on "Statistical inference and Monte Carlo algorithms," by G. Casella. *Test* **5**, 300-303.

Hastings, W.K. (1970). Monte Carlo sampling methods using Markov chains and their applications. *Biometrika* **57**, 97-109.

Hobert, J.P. and Casella, G. (1996). The effect of improper priors on Gibbs sampling in hierarchical linear mixed models. *Journal of the American Statistical Association* **91**, 1461-1473.

Hui, S.L. and Walter, S.D. (1980). Estimating the error rates of diagnostic tests. *Biometrics* **36**, 167-171.

Irwig, L.M., Groeneveld, H.T., and Simpson, J.M. (1990). Correcting for measurement error in an exposure-response relationship based on dichotomising a continuous dependent variable. *Australian Journal of Statistics* **32**, 261-269.

Iversen, Jr., E. S., Parmigiani, G., and Berry, D. (1999). Validating Bayesian prediction models: a case study in genetic susceptibility to breast cancer. In *Case Studies In Bayesian Statistics, Volume IV* (C. Gatsonis, R.E. Kass, B.P. Carlin, A. Carriquiry, A. Gelman, I. Verdinelli, and M. West, eds.). Springer, New York.

Johnson, W.O. and Gastwirth, J.L. (1991). Bayesian inference for medical screening tests: approximations useful for the analysis of acquired immune deficiency syndrome. *Journal of the Royal Statistical Society B* **53**, 427-439.

Johnson, W.O., Gastwirth, J.L., and Pearson, L.M. (2001). Screening without a "gold-standard": the Hui-Walter paradigm revisited. *American Journal of Epidemiology* **153**, 921-924.

Joseph, L., Gyorkos, T.W., and Coupal, L. (1995). Bayesian estimation of disease prevalence and the parameters of diagnostic tests in the absence of a gold standard. *American Journal of Epidemiology* **141**, 263-272.

Kadane, J.B. and Wolfson, L.J. (1998). Experiences in elicitation. *The Statistician* **47**, 3-19.

Kass, R.E. and Wasserman, L. (1995). A reference Bayesian test for nested hypotheses and its relationship to the Schwarz criterion. *Journal of the American Statistical Association* **90**, 928-934.

Ko, H. and Davidian, M. (2000). Correcting for measurement error in individual-level covariates in nonlinear mixed-effects models. *Biometrics* **56**, 368-375.

Kosinski, A.S. and Flanders, W.D. (1999). Evaluating the exposure and disease relationship with adjustment for different types of exposure misclassification: a regression approach. *Statistics in Medicine* **18**, 2795-2808.

Kuchenhoff, H. and Carroll, R.J. (1997). Segmented regression with errors in predictors: semiparametric and parametric methods. *Statistics in Medicine* **16**, 169-188.

Lagakos, S.W. (1988). Effects of mismodelling and mismeasuring explanatory variables on tests of their association with a response variable. *Statistics in Medicine* **7**, 257-274.

Lavine, M. (1992). Some aspects of Pólya tree distributions for statistical modelling. *Annals of Statistics* **20**, 1222-1235.

Liu, J.S. (2001). *Monte Carlo Strategies in Scientific Computing.* Springer, New York.

Louis, T.A. (1982). Finding the observed information matrix when using the EM algorithm. *Journal of the Royal Statistical Society B* **44**, 226-233.

Lyles, R.H. and Kupper, L.L. (1997). A detailed evaluation of adjustment methods for multiplicative measurement error in linear regression with applications in occupational epidemiology. *Biometrics* **53**, 1008-1025.

Mallick, B., Hoffman, F.O., and Carroll, R.J. (2002). Semiparametric regression modelling with mixtures of Berkson and classical error, with application to fallout from the Nevada test site. *Biometrics* **58**, 13-20.

Mallick, B.K. and Gelfand, A.E. (1996). Semiparametric errors in variables models: a Bayesian approach. *Journal of Statistical Planning and Inference* **52**, 307-321.

Mengersen, K.L, Robert, C.P., and Guihenneuc-Jouyaux, C. (1999). MCMC convergence diagnostics: a reviewww. In *Bayesian Statistics 6* (J.M. Bernardo, J.O. Berger, A.P. Dawid, and A.F.M. Smith, eds.). Oxford University Press, Oxford.

Metropolis, N., Rosenbluth, A.W., Rosenbluth, M.N., Teller, A.H., and Teller, E. (1953). Equations of state calculations by fast computing machines. *Journal of Chemical Physics* **21**, 1087-1092.

Morrissey, M.J. and Spiegelman, D. (1999). Matrix methods for estimating odds ratios with misclassified exposure data: extensions and comparisons. *Biometrics* **55**, 338-344.

Muller, P. and Roeder, K. (1997). A Bayesian semiparametric model for case-control studies with errors in variables. *Biometrika* **84**, 523-537.

Neath, A.E. and Samaniego, F.J. (1997). On the efficacy of Bayesian inference for nonidentifiable models. *American Statistician* **51**, 225-232.

O'Hagan, A. (1998). Eliciting expert beliefs in substantial practical applications. *The Statistician* **47**, 21-35.

Prentice, R.L. and Pyke, R. (1979). Logistic disease incidence models and case-control studies. *Biometrika* **66**, 403-411.

Richardson, S. and Gilks, W.R. (1993a). A Bayesian approach to measurement error problems in epidemiology using conditional independence models. *American Journal of Epidemiology* **138**, 430-442.

Richardson, S. and Gilks, W.R. (1993b). Conditional independence models for epidemiological studies with covariate measurement error. *Statistics in Medicine* **12**, 1703-1722.

Richardson, S. and Green, P.J. (1997). On Bayesian analysis of mixtures with an unknown number of components (with discussion). *Journal of the Royal Statistical Society B* **59**, 731-792.

Richardson, S. and Leblond, L. (1997). Some comments on misspecification of priors in Bayesian modelling of measurement error problems. *Statistics in Medicine* **16**, 203-213.

Richardson, S., Leblond, L., Jaussent, I., and Green, P.J. (2002). Mixture models in measurement error problems, with reference to epidemiological studies. *Journal of the Royal Statistical Society A* **165**, 549-566.

Ríos Insua, D. and Ruggeri, F. (eds.) (2000). *Robust Bayesian Analysis*. Springer, New York.

Robert, C.P. and Casella, G. (1999). *Monte Carlo Statistical Methods*. Springer, New York.

Roberts, G.O., Gelman, A., and Gilks, W.R. (1997). Weak convergence and optimal scaling of random walk Metropolis algorithms. *Annals of Applied Probability* **7**, 110-120.

Roberts, G.O. and Rosenthal, J.S. (2001). Optimal scaling for various Metropolis Hastings algorithms. *Statistical Science* **16**, 351-367.

Roberts, G.O. and Sahu, S.K. (1997). Updating schemes, correlation structure, blocking and parameterization for the Gibbs sampler. *Journal of the Royal Statistical Society B* **59**, 291-317.

Roeder, K., Carroll, R.J., and Lindsay, B.G. (1996). A semiparametric mixture approach to case-control studies with errors in covariables. *Journal of the American Statistical Association* **91**, 722-732.

Rosner, B. and Gore, R. (2001). Measurement error correction in nutritional epidemiology based on individual foods, with application to the relation of diet to breast cancer. *American Journal of Epidemiology* **154**, 827-835.

Rosner, B., Spiegelman, D., and Willett, W.C. (1990). Correction of logistic regression relative risk estimates and confidence intervals for measurement error: the case of multiple covariates measured with error. *American Journal of Epidemiology* **132**, 734-745.

Rosner, B., Willett, W.C., and Spiegelman, D. (1989). Correction of logistic regression relative risk estimates and confidence intervals for systematic within-person measurement error. *Statistics in Medicine* **8**, 1051-1070.

Schafer, D.W. (1987). Covariate measurement error in generalized linear models. *Biometrika* **74**, 385-391.

Seaman, S.R. and Richardson, S. (2001). Bayesian analysis of case-control studies with categorical covariates. *Biometrika* **88**, 1073-1088.

Schmid, C.H. and Rosner, B. (1993). A Bayesian approach to logistic regression models having measurement error following a mixture distribution. *Statistics in Medicine* **12**, 1141-1153.

Silverman, B.W. (1986). *Density Estimation for Statistics and Data Analysis*. Chapman and Hall, Boca Raton.

Spiegelman, D. (1994). Cost-efficient study designs for relative risk modelling with covariate measurement error. *Journal of Statistical Planning and Inference* **42**, 187-208.

Stefanski, L.A. and Carroll, R.J. (1985). Covariate measurement error in logistic regression. *Annals of Statistics* **13**, 1335-1351.

Stephens, D.A. and Dellaportas, P. (1992). Bayesian analysis of generalised linear models with covariate measurement error. In *Bayesian Statistics 4* (J.M.

Bernardo, J.O. Berger, A.P. Dawid, and A.F.M. Smith, eds.). Oxford University Press, Oxford.

Thomas, D., Stram, D. and Dwyer, J. (1993). Exposure measurement error: influence on exposure-disease relationships and methods of correction. *Annual Review of Public Health* **14**, 69-93.

Torrance-Rynard, V.L. and Walter, S.D. (1997). Effects of dependent errors in the assessment of diagnostic test performance *Statistics in Medicine* **16**, 2157-2175.

Tu, X.M., Kowalski, J., and Jia, G. (1999). Bayesian analysis of prevalence with covariates using simulation-based techniques: applications to HIV screening. *Statistics in Medicine* **18**, 3059-3073.

Vacek, P.M. (1985). The effect of conditional dependence on the evaluation of diagnostic tests. *Biometrics* **41**, 959-968.

Viana, M.A.G. (1994). Bayesian small-sample estimation of misclassified multinomial data. *Biometrics* **50**, 237-243.

Viana, M.A.G. and Ramakrishnan, V. (1992). Bayesian estimates of predictive value and related parameters of a diagnostic test. *Canadian Journal of Statistics* **20**, 311-321.

Walter, S.D. and Irwig, L.M. (1987). Estimation of test error rates, disease prevalence and relative risk from misclassified data: a review. *Journal of Clinical Epidemiology* **41**, 923-937.

Weinberg, C.R., Umbach, D.M., and Greenland, S. (1994). When will nondifferential misclassification of an exposure preserve the direction of a trend? (with discussion) *American Journal of Epidemiology* **140**, 565-571.

White, H. (1982). Maximum likelihood estimation of misspecified models. *Econometrika* **50**, 1-26.

Willett, W. (1989). An overview of issues related to the correction of nondifferential exposure measurement error in epidemiologic studies. *Statistics in Medicine* **8**, 1031-1040.

Wu, H. and Ding, A.A. (1999). Population HIV-1 dynamics *in vivo*: applicable models and inferential tools for virological data from AIDS clinical trials. *Biometrics* **55**, 410-418.

Wu, L. (2002). A joint model for nonlinear mixed-effects models with censoring and covariates measured with error, with application to AIDS studies. *Journal of the American Statistical Association* **97**, 955-964.

Wynder E.L. and Hoffman D. (1982). Tobacco. In *Cancer Epidemiology and Prevention* (D. Schottenfeld and J.K. Fraumeni Jr., eds.). WB Saunders, Philadelphia. pp. 277-292.

Zidek, J.V., Wong, H., Le, N.D., and Burnett, R. (1996). Causality, measurement error and collinearity in epidemiology. *Environmetrics* **7**, 441-451.

Index

accentuation, 47, 49
adjusting with false certainty, 107, 161
adjusting with uncertainty, 107
attenuation, 5
    curve, 11
    factor, 10
    realized, 22

bias versus variance, 104, 154, 161
biochemical variable, 2
bladder cancer, 69

caffeine, 1
case-control study, 69, 99, 111
collapsed model, 62
conditional exposure model, 54
confounding, 13
coronary artery disease, 122
credible interval, 110, 169

decision theory, 168
dichotomized variable, 139, 149
differential mismeasurement, 26, 124,
    142
    in case-control study, 46–47
Dirichlet distribution, 80, 135
dual exposure assessment, 111, 162
    in three populations, 126
    with dependence, 114, 124

EM algorithm, 52, 89, 114
exposure
    assessment, 3
    examples of, 1–3
    model, 52
    rare, 37, 39
exposure given outcome model, 120

flexible model, 74, 79–83

Framingham study, 72
full conditional distribution, 92, 171

Gibbs sampler, 58, 112, 127, 131, 171
grid-based model, 79

half-Cauchy distribution, 65
hyperparameter, 166

identifiability, 54–55, 108, 126, 152
importance sampling, 86
independence MH algorithm, 94
indirect learning, 154
inverse gamma distribution, 176

laboratory assay, 3
logistic regression, 24, 44, 69, 94, 123
    pseudo-equations, 25, 33

Markov chain Monte Carlo, 169–171
    acceptance rate, 173
    convergence, 58, 170
    mixing, 58, 170
    output analysis, 175
    simulation error, 175
measurement model, 52
mixed effects model, 62
model misspecification, 74, 77, 79, 147
multiple mismeasurement, 18
multiplicative mismeasurement, 15, 70

naive estimation, 3
nondifferential mismeasurement, 10
nutritional study, 2

odds-ratio, 39
outcome model, 52